2008

DR. FRED

AND THE

SPANISH LADY

DR. FRED

AND THE

SPANISH LADY

FIGHTING THE KILLER FLU

BETTY O'KEEFE AND IAN MACDONALD

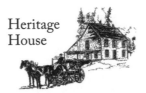

Heritage
House

This book is dedicated to the memory of the many courageous and self-sacrificing doctors, nurses, health-care workers, and volunteers in Canada who, sadly, gave their lives tending to the needs of those stricken by the 1918 Spanish flu.

National Library of Canada Cataloguing in Publication

O'Keefe, Betty, 1930-
    Dr. Fred and the Spanish lady: fighting the killer flu/Betty O'Keefe and Ian Macdonald.

Includes bibliographical references and index.
ISBN 1-894384-71-7

    1. Underhill, Fred. 2. Influenza—British Columbia—Vancouver—History—20th century. 3. Public health—British Columbia—Vancouver—History—20th century. I. Macdonald, Ian, 1928-   II. Title.

RC150.55.C32V36 2004   614.5'18'092   C2004-902307-1

First edition 2004

Heritage House acknowledges the financial support for our publishing program from the Government of Canada through the Book Publishing Industry Development Program (BPIDP), Canada Council for the Arts, and the British Columbia Arts Council.

Cover and book design by Nancy St.Gelais
Edited by Laurel Bernard and Vivian Sinclair

HERITAGE HOUSE PUBLISHING COMPANY LTD.
Unit #108 – 17665 66A Ave., Surrey, BC V3S 2A7

Printed in Canada

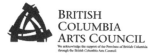

BRITISH
COLUMBIA
ARTS COUNCIL
We acknowledge the support of the Province of British Columbia
through the British Columbia Arts Council

The Canada Council | Le Conseil des Arts
for the Arts | du Canada

ACKNOWLEDGEMENTS

Particular thanks are extended to four members of the Underhill family—Richard Underhill and Mary Nicolls of Bowen Island, Helen Underhill of Vancouver, and Mark Underhill of Victoria—for sharing their photographs, letters, papers, and memories of Frederick and Beatrice Underhill. The quotes from Dr. Underhill that appear in this book come from these sources. The authors thank the following individuals for their assistance and cooperation during the preparation of this book:

Dr. Christofer Balram, Provincial Epidemiologist, New
    Brunswick
Deborah Scott Douglas, Canadian Medical Association,
    Ottawa
Dean Giustini, University of B.C. Biomedical Branch Library
Dr. John Blatherwick, Chief Medical Health Officer,
    Vancouver Coastal Health Authority
Dr. K. Grimsrud, Deputy Provincial Health Officer, Alberta
Melanie Hardbattle, St. Paul's Hospital Archives
Anna Hayes, Nicole Boucher, and Janet Lirenman, Lord
    Nelson School, Vancouver
Vera Lucas, Victoria
Sheena Macdonald, Vancouver
B. Rick MacLowick, Manitoba Legislative Library, Winnipeg
Leslie Myers, B.C. Nurses Association, Vancouver
Lamont Sweet, Chief Health Officer, Prince Edward Island

Dr. Theresa Tam, Department of Health and Welfare, Ottawa
Virginia Walden, VGH graduate, Tsawwassen
Ethel Warbinek, Vancouver General Hospital School of
    Nursing Alumnae
Sara Wotherspoon, B.C. College of Physicians and Surgeons

CONTENTS

FOREWORD

As this book went to press, the emergence of new flu strains continued to threaten human health around the world. In January 2004, an avian flu cropped up in southeast Asia, raising the fear of cross-species virus mutation to humans. The mysterious Severe Acute Respiratory Syndrome (SARS), which made its terrifying debut in 2003, remains a constant danger. In British Columbia, an atypical flu season in late 2003 included a new virulent strain that targeted children. In the early months of 2004, avian flu appeared in B.C.'s Fraser Valley, resulting in the killing of all poultry in the area and bringing the reality of new flu threats home to roost. The man leading Vancouver's public health battle is Chief Medical Health Officer Dr. John Blatherwick.

☆   ☆   ☆

Hanging in my office is a photograph of a man in whose footsteps I am proud to follow exactly 100 years later.

Dr. Frederick Theodore Underhill was the city's first full-time medical health officer and was a pioneer in public health in Vancouver. In 1904, some 10 years after he came to British Columbia from England and with the experience gained from medical practices in England, Mission, B.C., and Vancouver's West End, he gladly undertook the duties of medical health officer in the 18-year-old city.

From his first day on the job to his last, he pursued with unswerving dedication programs geared to improve the health of the public. He organized the first regular garbage collection. He helped push for improvements to the water supply and instituted better inspection of meats and other foodstuffs.

Vancouver at the beginning of the 20th century had one of the country's highest infant mortality rates. He changed that disturbing figure by setting up a baby clinic and in time established a record for the lowest infant mortality.

He was a 60-year-old man when the killer Spanish flu pandemic reached B.C. in 1918, killing some 4,400 people. But Dr. Fred Underhill's untiring, sure-handed direction helped guide Vancouver residents through the suffering and death that came with the disease. He was MHO for 26 years.

Nobody knows the importance of the contributions he made to improving Vancouver's public health better than those of us who followed him: Dr. J.W. McIntosh, 1930–1938; Dr. Stewart Murray, 1938–1960; Dr. Joe Gayton, 1960–1967; Dr. Gerry Bonham, 1967–1979; Dr. David Kinloch, 1979–1982; Dr. John Smith (Acting MHO), 1982–1984; and myself, 1984 to the present. As Gerry said to me when I took on the job, "Keep it, it's the best job you'll ever have."

In 2004, when new and alarming flu-type illnesses threaten the world, Fred Underhill's urging still rings true as a simple but effective weapon against the spread of disease: "Wash your hands well and frequently."

John Blatherwick, CM, CD, MD, FRCP(C)
Chief Medical Health Officer
Vancouver Coastal Health Authority
British Columbia, Canada
January 14, 2004

INTRODUCTION

"We really weren't under any medical supervision at all. It was all just guesswork. We tried to be as nice to them as we could and just be with them when they died."

When the world's worst pandemic invaded Canada in 1918, it struck with a deadly force never known before, swamping the country's meagre health resources. The words of courageous teenagers Lillian and Kay Estabrooks, who tended to the sick in the small mining community of Hedley, British Columbia, testify to the desperate situation faced by hundreds of young volunteers, doctors, and nurses across the country as they coped with the mysterious "Spanish flu." Battling a deadly and fast-moving enemy, they risked and often sacrificed their lives to relieve the suffering and horror of the victims.

The people of Canada were already doing their best to deal with sorrow and heartbreak, the results of World War I's terrible death toll. Home-front life was being played out against a backdrop of four years of the most destructive war in the world's history. Since the guns had first boomed on the Western Front in 1914, millions had been slaughtered, and by 1918, 60,000 Canadians lay dead in battlefields and oceans around the world.

Into this national tragedy came the flu, sweeping inexorably from the St. Lawrence to the Maritimes, Ontario, and the far reaches of the Prairies, and quickly arriving on the west coast. It was a pandemic—an epidemic that moved rapidly from one region to another, crossing national boundaries and jumping across oceans to new continents with ease. Most often called the Spanish flu or the Spanish Lady, this virus spared few parts of the world in a global sweep that killed many more than 25 million, and possibly as many as 50 million, of the earth's inhabitants.

Today's wonder drugs and advanced medical techniques were unknown when the Spanish Lady arrived, and doctors had little to aid them in the fight against a foe they had never encountered before. Hospital wards quickly overflowed, and schools, church halls, old hotels, and other facilities were pressed into service as isolation hospitals. Nurses garbed from head to toe in white gowns moved like apparitions through wards tightly packed with beds only inches apart. They watched helplessly as what began as flu often developed into pneumonia with fatal results. The world had lived with flu for centuries, but this was a new killer strain.

In many communities, schools, places of entertainment, meeting halls, and even churches were closed. Thousands were sick and dying; families grieved; new, previously unheard-of laws and health restrictions were enforced; factories, forests, and mines curtailed production as workers were stricken; and everyday life became more difficult and, for some, unbearable.

Daily funeral processions wound their mournful way through city streets, and similar scenes were repeated in every town, village, and hamlet across the country. Gravediggers worked long hours into the night and still couldn't fill the demand. Flowers for wreaths were in short supply. Often, people wore masks when they walked the streets. Some people took refuge at home, refusing to associate with others, answer the door, or go out; often, the flu found them anyway.

From its early appearance in eastern Canada in mid-1918, the pandemic lingered in Canada for about 18 months, peaking in the fall of the year. There was no cure, and before it had run its course, 50,000 Canadians from a population of eight million joined the ranks of those who had already perished in the trenches of western Europe and on the high seas.

When the flu finally faded away, medical scientists around the world still knew little about it and had failed to identify why it took so many lives. Canada, in an average year, loses about 1,400 people to common outbreaks of the flu. Recent viral outbreaks may be harbingers of worse episodes to come in the future; microbiologists warn that another pandemic is overdue and that it could be just as lethal as the 1918 variety, if not worse.

The most frightening outbreak since 1918 was the notorious Hong Kong flu of 1997. Highly infectious, the flu carried within it the potential to kill millions upon millions of people. As the Spanish flu is believed to have done, it jumped the species barrier from animal to human. Moving from chickens to people, the Hong Kong flu killed relatively few humans, but only because alert officials ordered the slaughter of all the chickens on the island of Hong Kong in time to stop it.

Another chicken flu with the same deadly potential surfaced in Vietnam in January 2004 and quickly spread to other nearby countries. The slaughter of millions of chickens followed. Fortunately, in the early stages the flu was transmitted only from chicken to chicken and occasionally from chicken to human, so the number of people who died in the first few months of the year was not large. Each viral outbreak of this type, however, has the potential to develop into another worldwide pandemic, the virus mutating so that it can be passed from human to human and then spreading like wildfire through the population. Many scientists predict that the next pandemic will originate in the near future in southeast Asia.

Severe Acute Respiratory Syndrome, better known as SARS, struck Canada without warning in 2003, killing 44 people in the first half of the year from a population of 30 million. The estimated mortality rate of the Spanish flu was 2.5 percent worldwide, while SARS' toll—with 8,500 cases and 800 deaths as of July 2003—was three times higher than that. There were more than 150 cases in Canada, almost all of them in Toronto, the most seriously affected area outside of Asia.

Despite advances in medical science since 1918 and such institutions as the World Health Organization, it was still difficult to halt the spread of SARS once it had taken hold. Toronto's early cases went undetected, allowing the disease to spread widely among families and health-care workers. Vancouver, under the leadership of such health authorities as Vancouver Coastal Health Officer Dr.

John Blatherwick and Dr. Robert C. Burnham, medical director of the B.C. Centre for Disease Control, fared better. The outbreak was detected early, victims were isolated, and health-care workers were protected.

In 1918 there were far fewer resources available to health-care professionals than there are today. There was no organization in Canada to show leadership and direct the counter-attack. Today there is Health Canada with its national monitoring system and a special section that deals strictly with immunization and respiratory infections. The major cities of Canada were much smaller in 1918 than they are today, and each one relied largely on its own medical health officer and health-care workers to deal with infectious diseases. In Charlottetown, Halifax, Montreal, Toronto, Winnipeg, Regina, Saskatoon, Edmonton, Calgary, Vancouver, and Victoria, the fight was carried on by doctors, nurses, hospital matrons, and boards of health who laboured 24 hours a day in an attempt to keep people alive.

What scant information that was available on how to fight the disease came from doctors in cities around the world who had already struggled while patients lay dying around them. They were medical practitioners in London, Berlin, Capetown, and even Beijing (then known as Peking). Doctors in Canada sought out their contemporaries in New York, Boston, Seattle, San Francisco, and at the Mayo Clinic in Rochester, Minnesota, for suggestions and advice. Whether it was a man responsible for the health of a country, like Britain's Dr. George Newman in London, or a young woman like Dr. Isobel Arthur, the health officer for the small town of Nelson, B.C., they were all locked in the same struggle.

These are the people who held the line on a city-by-city, town-by-town, village-by-village basis in lonely struggles from Atlantic to Pacific. There were many unsung heroes who toiled in obscurity until they dropped. There were also individuals who emerged on the public scene in the right place at the right time and carried the day. On Canada's west coast, one of these was Dr. Frederick Theodore Underhill, Vancouver's first full-time public health officer. At the age of 60, as the pandemic finally consumed the entire continent, he was the man who led the charge and developed the tactics for survival.

18

The story of the Spanish flu in Canada and Underhill's encounter with the deadly señora is a tribute to doctors, nurses, and caregivers everywhere. His knowledge and dedication were matched in many other centres, where co-operation and a common goal brought out the best in the medical profession. It is a story of individuals, their experiences, their fears, their worries, suffering, heroism, and sacrifice. Some used common sense and innovation, others panicked, and there was often confusion about what to do. But overall, a spirit of co-operation and compassion developed within cities and towns that saved many lives from one of humankind's most implacable and persistent enemies.

TIMELINE FOR SPANISH FLU

Mid-1917: Reports emerge of a mysterious killer, a flu-like illness originating in China and sweeping Asia and Eastern Europe.

Early 1918: Canadian and other troops fighting the First World War in France are ravaged by a new disease.

Doctors are confronted by a lethal flu strain never known before that strikes and spreads quickly.

March 1918: Canadian military and government representatives meet to plan facilities for expected soldier victims of what is now recognized as a pandemic.

Spring: Flu sweeps through congested U.S. army camps, leaving many dead. There are heavy civilian victims in Boston and other cities.

September: Infected returning soldiers land at Quebec City, bringing flu to Canada; first civilian cases are at a Victoriaville school.

Within days thousands are sick and dying in Montreal and other Quebec communities.

The disease spreads rapidly into the Maritime Provinces, Ontario, and the West, carried partly by infected soldiers on trains going home.

Early October: The disease arrives in B.C., with many victims in Kootenay mining towns. Officials close schools and entertainment centres in most towns and villages.

Victoria and Vancouver hospitals are swamped, the latter by many sick coming from nearby communities with no medical facilities. Gravediggers are in short supply.

October 18: Vancouver's medical health officer, Dr. Frederick Underhill, orders schools and entertainment centres closed, Victoria having done so earlier. In both cities commercial and industrial plants remain open.

Civic leaders make urgent pleas for volunteers to help nurse the sick and dying. Vancouver victims now number in the thousands.

October 27: Vancouver's worst day, 24 dead within 24 hours; flu ravaging coastal and interior communities.

November 11: People forget worries about the flu and flock into the streets to celebrate the end of World War One.

November 19: Dr. Underhill orders city reopened as flu begins to abate. Victoria follows suit.

Province's top medical man, Provincial Health Officer Dr. Henry Young, says records are incomplete and at times inaccurate, but estimates the Spanish flu pandemic of 1918–early 1919 took the lives of some 4,400 British Columbians.

A CENTURIES-OLD KILLER

Influenza is an Italian word that came into being following an epidemic in 1504, when it was believed that the disease was caused by the influence of the stars. In a later age it was dubbed *influenza di friddo*, meaning "influence of the cold." When it appeared in 1918, influenza became "the Spanish flu" or "the Spanish Lady," a misnomer coined because initial press reports about it originated in Spain. Once the virus reached Great Britain, it was called Flanders Grippe; in Hungary, it was the Black Whip; in Japan, they called it Wrestlers' Fever; to the Persians it was the Disease of the Wind; the Poles dubbed it the Bolshevik Disease; the Swiss called it the Coquette; and to the Germans, it was Blitz Katarrh—Lightning Cold. In any language, it brought severe sickness, pain, and death to millions of people.

Ever since detailed medical documentation began to be kept in diaries and letters, possibly as early as 400 BC in the writings of Hippocrates and Livy, an erratic recurrence of this disease has been evident. Medical historians have detected differences in flu epidemics, and how they affected people living in various countries at different times.

Scientists are confident it was an outbreak of the flu that was graphically and dramatically described some 450 years ago in a letter to Lord Cecil from Lord Randolph. He wrote of an attack suffered by Mary, Queen of Scots while in Edinburgh:

Maye it please your Honor, immediately upon
the Quene's [Mary's] arrival here, she fell
acquainted with a new disease that is common in
this towne, called here the newe acquayntance,
which passed also throughe her whole courte,
neither sparinge lordes, ladies nor damoysells
not so much as 'ether Frenche or English. It ys a
plague in their heades that have yt, and a sorenes
in their stomackes, with a great coughe, that
remayneth with some longer, with others shorter
tyme, as yt findeth apte bodies for the nature
of the disease. The quene kept her bed six days.
There was no appearance of danger, nor manie
that die of the disease, excepte some olde folkes.
My Lord Murraye is now presently in it, the
lord of Lidlington hathe had it, and I ashamed
to say that I have byne free of it, seinge it seketh
acquayntance at all men's handes.

The letter points out that the death toll in this epidemic was not
great, although Lord Randolph's "excepte some olde folkes" may be
misleading. In the mid-16th century, the age of 40 was considered
quite old, and Randolph may also have overlooked a few deaths in
his casual disregard for the senior citizens of his age.

Flu outbreaks continued through succeeding centuries. There
is considerable information about a flu pandemic that occurred in
1742–43 and resulted in widespread European outbreaks. In Rome
80,000 were reported ill, with 500 buried in one day. Italy was ravaged
by flu again in 1781–82, and at the same time, St. Petersburg in
Russia reported 30,000 were ill. South America had an outbreak in
1801. Russia was said to be the starting point for an onslaught of the
disease in 1847–48, when almost half of Paris was sick and London
reported 7,000 deaths in six weeks. This was indeed a pandemic,
affecting many countries and several continents, even reaching as far
away as Australia in 1850.

Germans were felled by the thousands in another onslaught that
struck mid-Europe in 1889–90. It was the last and the most severe

of six waves of the disease recorded in the 19th century. Before the strain ran its course, it killed 250,000 people in Europe.

Researchers now believe that the Spanish flu of 1918 originated in China, like SARS, and first appeared in the province of Guangdong. From there, it seems to have reached Canton, China's big trading port, where there were reports of a serious, rapidly spreading sickness. It then moved into eastern and central Europe, carried by travellers on boats and in trains, and there it found a continent weakened by war.

Spain got the blame for the flu because as a neutral country in World War One, its newspapers were not censored and first reports of a widespread epidemic appeared in stories published in Barcelona and Madrid. By then the whole of Europe was feeling the wrath of the Spanish Lady.

The extent of her assault on Asia remains largely undocumented, but it is known that she decimated the allied armies in Europe, as well as the opposing forces of Germany. She may even have helped hasten the end of the conflict because so many soldiers were ill that it was at times difficult to carry on. Ailing North American troops were invalided home from the war in the trenches suffering from the effects of poison gas; bullet, bayonet, and shrapnel wounds; and a mysterious, severe, often fatal type of flu.

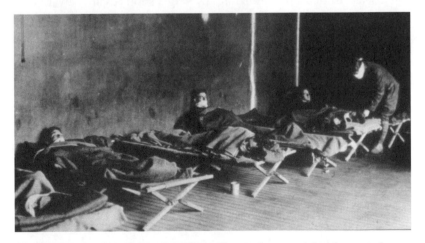

The Spanish flu of 1918 was first felt in Europe, by troops already worn down by the war. Pictured here is an influenza ward in U.S. Army Field Hospital No. 29, in Hollerich, Luxembourg.

The same applied to the armies of other nations as they headed home. Russia was in particularly dire straits following the collapse of its war against Germany and the 1917 Bolshevik revolution. In many European countries there had been years of food shortages and malnutrition, leaving populations generally in poor health, easy prey for any disease. Perhaps this was a factor that contributed to the severity of the pandemic. In any case, as the war neared its end, a new death-dealing assault on the peoples of every land began, one that would claim more lives than did the four long years of war.

Characteristics of the flu

The Spanish flu started like a regular wintertime complaint. There was a cough, a sore throat, and a runny nose, accompanied by fever and body aches and pains. Most of those who caught it were forced into their beds. Tragically—and inexplicably—it was the young and the healthy, the ones most likely to tough it out, who were felled by the terrifying malady.

The flu seemed to become more severe as it crossed countries and continents, developing into a sudden, ferocious type of pneumonia that brought death, often within hours. Doctors, although they found the disease difficult to combat at any stage, soon became aware that if a patient developed pneumonia, it would prove fatal 40 percent of the time.

Medical men in England reported that just before dying their patients often turned an odd shade of blue, which they described as heliotrope cyanosis. In the United States, doctors said some patients turned a deep brown before they died, making it difficult to tell if the deceased was "white or coloured." In Labrador, some sufferers became dark red. Often, doctors wondered if they were dealing with a new form of typhus or cholera. Some even compared the severity of the disease to the Black Death, the bubonic plague that killed a quarter of Europe's population in the 14th century.

Over the course of history, flu has been blamed on everything from the positioning of the planets to earthquakes, volcanic eruptions, and the unhappiness of the gods. Only in more scientific times has the Spanish flu been blamed on a virus.

In 1892, the efforts of 19th-century scientists studying the flu virus were rewarded when Dr. Frederick Pfeiffer, head of the Berlin Institute of Infectious Diseases, announced a partial breakthrough. Using specimens from the throats of sufferers, he had isolated the bacterium responsible for what he called *homophilus influenzae*. Known as Pfeiffer's bacillus, it was not then categorized as a virus. At this time, the differences between bacteria and viruses were not recognized. It wasn't until the 1930s that influenza viruses were isolated and cultured.

As always, another school of thought took an opposing position to the discovery, claiming that the German scientist had not identified the right bacillus. Meanwhile, Pfeiffer's findings attracted the attention of other specialists and sent them off in new directions in pursuit of new answers to how the disease developed, grew, and spread, and how it could be stopped.

As the Spanish Lady decimated Europe, allied military medical men desperately searched for effective treatment. Their investigations showed that the high mortality rate was due to a secondary invasion of the sick by "streptococcus pyogenes longus." Gradually, diagnosticians also identified differences between this epidemic and ones they had studied previously. A baffling aspect was the age of the victims. Previously, severe flu attacks had taken a heavy toll amongst the elderly and the very young, but this onslaught was attacking and killing those in their prime, people aged 20 to 40, and it affected more men than women—sometimes with an awful suddenness. This was one of the reasons why the armed forces overseas were so affected.

The deadly strain continued to baffle medical professionals globally. Even the military doctors stated that "no specific treatment was discovered" despite their best efforts. For those afflicted, there was no means of prevention, no effective treatment, and little that could be done to ease the symptoms.

In 1918 there were no sulpha drugs, no penicillin, or any of the other mid-20th-century antibiotics that have tamed such diseases as diphtheria and scarlet fever. Even Aspirin in tablet form was fairly new and was not in widespread use. During this pandemic, victims' temperatures often quickly soared to 104 degrees. Patients complained that they were freezing, despite the number of blankets piled on top of them and the roaring fires that turned homes into sweatboxes. There seemed to be no way to keep the seriously ill warm or to bring down the raging fevers from which they suffered. Those afflicted were often delirious, their bodies racked with pain, their chests congested. Dehydration followed as they gasped for air and slipped into semi-consciousness. As the disease spread it gained momentum, constantly mutating, so that some newly infected patients died within hours of exhibiting the first signs of sickness. Such ongoing change in symptoms was one of the signs that the disease was a virus, rather than a bacterial infection.

As the pandemic spread throughout the world, exhausted nurses and doctors found they could do nothing but apply cold compresses or slap on boiling hot-mustard plasters and wait for the fever to break. At home, families turned to old herbal remedies such as violet leaf or chamomile tea, ground garlic buds, sulphur and molasses tonic, or other home cures handed down from their grandparents.

In the public health field, there were early attempts to produce vaccines, but these serums were of questionable worth. Most were a mixture of blood and mucus taken from infected people; the most visible result was a badly infected arm for those who received the treatment.

Spanish flu's killing power

Statisticians have had great difficulty confirming the actual number of victims from the pandemic of 1918. Throughout the world, records have been lost, were never kept, or are so sketchy that it is likely many more people died than was reported. Official figures in countries like China, India, other Asian nations, and Russia were poor, speculation at best. In Europe, it was often impossible to separate the war dead from the flu dead.

Many epidemiologists contend that the death toll might easily have been twice the 25 million sometimes cited, possibly between 40 and 50 million people. A few have even speculated that 100 million people died worldwide. No matter what the toll, it is a devastating figure, especially when one remembers that early in the 20th century the world's population was much smaller, making the proportion of people killed by the flu truly appalling.

By early 1918 the Spanish Lady had already thrown her shadow across the Atlantic Ocean, but few in Canada were yet aware of her existence. Those who remained at home—wives, mothers, fathers, grandparents, relatives, and friends—had become reluctant to read newspapers because they feared what they might find. As a consequence, many missed the significance of a front-page headline that appeared in the Toronto *Globe and Mail* midway through the year: "Flanders Grippe Spreads in Foe Ranks. Whole Divisions Are Stricken With The Sneezing Illness." Moreover, at this stage most people believed it was just another outbreak of the flu, maybe a little more serious than usual.

The news story suggested that this illness was the reason for recent relatively scaled-down activity along the front line in France. Reportedly, the Germans had been forced to pull two battalions out of the trenches because of the number of sick soldiers. There was speculation that the flu had hit both sides in France, and consequently there had been less fighting in recent months in many sectors, with fewer casualties than expected. The slaughter was so great, however, and had continued for so long, that "light" losses for one week, reported by the British in September, meant 432 officers and 3,926 men killed, and 20,000 reported wounded or missing.

The story also stated that it would have been almost impossible for the mighty British home fleet to sail into action in May because more than 10,000 sailors were sick. One of Canada's artillery units had been similarly decimated by illness.

Meanwhile, newspapers were running long lists of Canadian casualties at least once each week, sometimes more. Canadians had become accustomed to seeing black-boxed, single-column pictures of men they knew or might have come to know, teenagers, brothers, and fathers who "Paid the Supreme Sacrifice," "Fell for Their Country," or "Met a Gallant End." The lists often filled many columns and included the names of men killed by disease, along with the missing, those believed to be prisoners of war, and those who had died of wounds. One prominent Canadian who caught the flu and died of pneumonia in France was Colonel John McCrae, the surgeon-poet who wrote "In Flanders Fields." There were thousands of others.

Troopships continued to transport fresh recruits to Europe before returning home with beds full of the latest casualties—the wounded and the sick. The suffering of these men was not always relieved as the crowded vessels slowly ploughed their way home. For two weeks the victims of the war had to contend with turbulent seas and seasickness, and by the summer more and more were also being felled by the flu. Limited shipboard medical facilities were strained to the limit caring for the increasing number of soldiers forced into bed with flu symptoms during the voyage home. Officers gave up their cabins for use as small hospital wards, and sick soldiers were accommodated wherever a cot could be squeezed in.

Ships regularly stopped in mid-Atlantic to perform solemn last rites for a great many men who had hoped they were finally returning home. Increasingly they were not dying from war wounds, but from the flu. While comrades watched in sombre silence, chaplains conducted full military funerals before canvas-covered bodies were

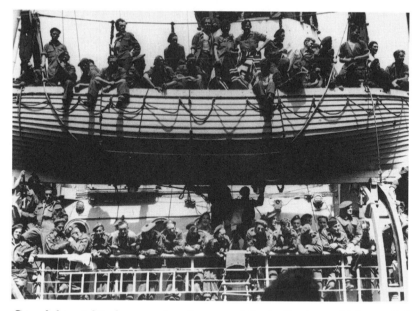

Crowded troopships became a breeding ground for the flu virus, which travelled in both directions. Canadian regiments like the Calgary Highlanders, seen here, unknowingly brought the disease home from the war.

slid into the cold sea and the sound of a bugle playing "The Last Post" echoed across the blackness of the waves.

By October 1918, every ship in Convoy HX50 had its flag at half-mast; two of them, the *Otranto* and *Kashmir*, collided, at least partly because many of the men operating the ships were ill. It was these troopships that were unwittingly bringing a new horror home to Canada. The returning troops who recovered or survived long enough to disembark in Quebec played an unfortunate but major role in escorting the Spanish Lady on her deadly dance across the continent.

A WAR-WEARY COUNTRY

The toll in the trenches of Flanders Fields had sapped much of the spirit of Canadians at home. They did not suffer the stark fate of so many in the battlefields of Europe, but they were nonetheless tired of rationing, shortages, and the sorrows of death. Everyone was war-weary. Almost every family had lost a son, a father, a brother, a daughter serving overseas as a nurse, a close friend, or a neighbour. Families often lost two, three, or four young men.

Typical of the reports seen daily in newspapers was one in Vancouver that read: "Brothers John and Alec Price, whose parents live on Prince Albert Street, were killed on the same day in France. They were beautiful in their lives and in death not divided." Lieutenant Alec Campbell-Johnson, who enlisted at the age of 15, and his brother Ronald met a similar fate. They were hailed as a "splendid type of Canadian youth."

Often it had seemed that a ceasefire was just around the corner, but hopes of peace had been dashed over and over again. Now Canada was on the brink of a new tragedy and no one was ready for it. No one could have envisioned quite how terrible it would be.

The national scene

Members of the Canadian military and the federal government knew the Spanish flu was coming. They feared that the illness, which had appeared south of the border on March 11, 1918, and was known to be ravaging much of Asia and Europe, would find its way to Canada and severely impact the country's ability to participate in the war. As a result, representatives of the various departments that would be involved in fighting a flu pandemic, should it arrive, gathered for a meeting in Ottawa on March 20.

Attending were personnel from public works, engineering, and medical services. They were informed that the military wanted to acquire additional hospitals from Charlottetown to Victoria as treatment facilities for returning soldiers. Many veterans were wounded, but the death toll from the flu was climbing, and the military was responsible for providing proper care for all no matter what the ailment. Already, they were having difficulty finding beds for the sick and dying soldiers, and they knew it was going to get worse.

Military plans moved forward quickly after the meeting—during a war, military expenditures always come first—but no group existed to coordinate national health concerns for the general public, a deficiency that was to become starkly clear in the coming months. No preparations outside the military were made before the Spanish Lady arrived; consequently, the fight against her more resembled guerrilla

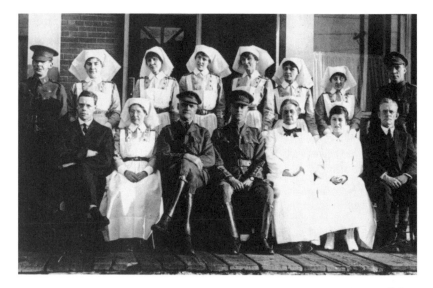

Staff at military hospitals were the first to tackle the flu.

sorties than a coordinated attack. Across the country, it was unclear who was responsible for what, but ingenuity and the belief that man should help his fellow man prevailed nearly everywhere.

The Pacific coast in 1918

Wartime Vancouver was full of shipyards and crammed with wartime workers. Over 5,000 were employed in the bustling yards of the waterfront, helping to meet wartime naval demands. Conditions in Seattle and San Francisco were equally hectic as servicemen and naval-yard shipbuilders toiled through the day and night to beat the Kaiser. In the U.S., however, rationing and shortages were not yet severe, as the nation had been at war for little more than a year.

The influx of people to Vancouver in the four years since the war had started had escalated the demand for everything from health services to accommodation. There was a shortage of housing, and conditions in many rooming houses were squalid. The war also had taken many local doctors and nurses to far-flung war fronts.

Whether residents of the U.S. or Canada, all those working on the home front flocked regularly to movie theatres and were happy to pay 10 cents to see silent flicks starring Charlie Chaplin, Canada's own Mary Pickford, Fatty Arbuckle, and William S. Hart in a variety of comedies, dramas, and westerns. Hart played Shark Munro, "the hard-fisted captain of an Alaskan sailing schooner." There was also William Fornum in *True Blue*, "a big vital drama of the plains about cowpunchers in Arizona and a man who abandoned an earldom for the only girl he loved."

For many people in Vancouver the pictures were not only entertainment, but also an opportunity to escape the overcrowded, damp, and drafty rooms they rented. Finding a tradesman to do repairs or build new housing was almost impossible. For four years there had been little time for anything except trying to win the war. The big old residences, the only housing available for single men and women, were sometimes without reliable plumbing or other amenities and were perfect breeding grounds for infectious diseases of all kinds. Often, there was only one bath in the house, shared by all the roomers.

Amongst the young, the feeling was that the less time spent at home, the better. Besides, on a day off, matinee-goers could treat themselves to a 40-cent lunch at Vancouver's Hudson's Bay store restaurant, selecting from a menu of cracked crab, beef, lamb, or pork and, as they ate, listening to the musical stylings of John Harvey's Orchestra.

Rural B.C. in 1918 contained many of the place names that remain familiar today, but the population was small. The vast majority of B.C.'s 440,000 inhabitants lived in the Lower Mainland and the Fraser River Valley, and there were only three cities of any size: Vancouver, with its more than 110,000 inhabitants and growing neighbour municipalities of Point Grey, South Vancouver, and Burnaby; Victoria, which had a population of about 38,000; and New Westminster, with 14,000 residents.

The rest of B.C. consisted of a series of smaller towns, such as Nanaimo, with a population of 9,000 including the surrounding area; Prince Rupert with 6,300 people; Nelson with 5,200; Kamloops with 4,500; and Fernie with 4,300. Other B.C. settlements were little more than villages, all of them home to fewer than 3,000 inhabitants. These included Trail, Revelstoke, Prince George, Kelowna, Cranbrook, and Port Alberni.

Hospitals and medical personnel were few and far between. Rural residents mostly fended for themselves. The people worked as homesteading farmers, miners, loggers, or shopkeepers catering to the needs of their contemporaries. Life was often rough and ready, but people in the small settlements made friends quickly and easily. They were all in the same boat, reliant in one way or another on each other, and when an emergency threatened, they pulled together to beat it.

The public health officers

In British Columbia, health authorities had some breathing space to gather what advice they could from outside sources. The disease ravaged much of North America before it struck the west coast. As it marched across the continent and made its way into the hinterland of B.C., three key people readied themselves for what they knew was to come. It was a struggle far worse than anything they had experienced previously or ever would again. These key medical men were Dr. Arthur Price, Victoria health officer; Dr. Henry Esson Young, provincial health officer; and Dr. Frederick Theodore Underhill, Vancouver health officer.

Arthur Price was born in 1863 and graduated from Trinity College, Dublin, in 1888. He registered with the College of Physicians and Surgeons of B.C. on November 3, 1910, and was appointed Victoria's medical health officer in 1917. He shared many of Underhill's views on public health, and the creation of a baby clinic in the capital was one of his early accomplishments.

Meticulous and precise in all his work but more youthful and less experienced than his two contemporaries, Price had only one objective: ensuring the good health of the people in his city. His brusque, often overbearing approach rubbed some people the wrong way, but in the end his methods proved most successful. He was a man with a lively mind, always ready to answer unquestioningly the call of King and Empire—to him the "British" in British Columbia said it all, very fitting for a Victorian of the time.

Price died in 1948 and was honoured in 1956 when a health and welfare centre in downtown Victoria was named after him. He was hailed as a pioneer of public health, and then-health minister Eric Martin said he was "a man who served his country and his community well indeed."

Dr. Henry Young, the province's top public health officer, strongly supported the need for preventive medicine, and a short-lived political career had taught him to be cautious in making public statements. Born in Quebec in 1867, Young was the son of a Scottish Presbyterian minister. He was a lean, craggy-featured man who acquired his medical degree from McGill University in Montreal and then studied in London, England, and in the United States. He also obtained a degree in geology, and it was this interest in mining and precious metals, along with a spirit of adventure, that brought him west. In 1903 he arrived in B.C., settling first at a new gold-mining camp in Atlin, a small, isolated community near the Yukon border.

Four years later he was talked into entering politics by Sir Richard McBride, who served as Conservative B.C. premier from 1903 to 1915. Young was elected as the member for Atlin on March

13, 1907, and became provincial secretary responsible for education and health.

After serving two terms in the Conservative cabinet, Young decided not to run for re-election in 1916, but gladly accepted the post of provincial health officer when it was offered to him. It gave him an opportunity to concentrate more fully on the field of medicine and to practise some of the things he had advocated during his terms in office. Within two years he would become embroiled in the most serious battle of his life. It was fortunate that the man who worked beside him was Dr. Frederick Underhill.

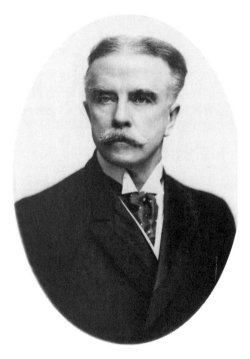

Dr. Henry Young was the senior provincial health officer at the time of the pandemic. The son of a Scottish Presbyterian minister, Young had a medical degree from McGill University and had studied in London, England, and in the United States.

DR. FREDERICK UNDERHILL

Adversity has a way of breeding heroes, and the 1918 pandemic was no exception. Towns, cities, and even nations are sometimes fortunate during times of great crisis to have the right person in the right place at the right time—someone with knowledge, dedication, unswerving confidence, and the willingness to take full responsibility. When the deadly Spanish flu swept into Vancouver, fate decreed that there would be such a person on hand. He was a courageous, innovative, young-thinking 60-year-old man, pioneer B.C. physician and public health officer Dr. Frederick Theodore Underhill.

Firm in his views, never overawed by authority, courteous but also tough, he had already won the title "guardian of Vancouver's public health." He was respected by both his peers and the public. He had worked closely with the provincial officer, Dr. Young, for nearly two years. They saw eye to eye on many issues affecting public health, and Young was fortunate to have such an experienced man in charge of the most heavily populated area of the province.

Born in Tipton, a town in Staffordshire in the English Midlands, on January 19, 1858, Fred Underhill was a member of a large family. He had five brothers, one sister, and two stepbrothers. His father, William Lees Underhill, and both of his grandfathers were physicians, so from childhood Fred's ambition was to be a doctor. When he completed his studies at Aldenham School at the age of 18, he began his career washing bottles and doing other menial chores for a local surgeon. However, at 20, he was able to enrol in Scotland's Edinburgh

University, graduating in 1881 and interning at the Royal Infirmary in Edinburgh. While attending college, he spent any time left over from his studies working for local physicians, and in 1885 he applied to be appointed as a medical officer.

The application required testimonials from prominent doctors in the region, and one of them wrote in glowing terms of young Dr. Underhill: "I have known him for some years past both personally and professionally and in both capacities know he is deservedly much liked and respected by all classes. His professional knowledge is extensive and his manner towards his patients is kindly and considerate."[1]

It was not long before Frederick met Beatrice, the daughter of a Tipton doctor. Beatrice Alice Muriel was a tiny woman, always ready for a new adventure, with a great zest for life and a fondness for gambling. Beatrice got all she could have asked for when she married Fred Underhill, including 13 children by him.

The new doctor spent his early years practising medicine in Tipton, tending to the ills and misfortunes of his friends and neighbours. He was also a surgeon in the volunteer battalion of the Fourth South Staffordshire Rifles, and in what remaining spare time he could find, he played cricket and tennis and was a keen gardener. His patients called him out at all hours of the day and night, and after several years of working long hours with too little rest, he became seriously ill. He explained, "I never had a holiday in England after I left school. The first holiday of my life I had to take, for my health had broken down, and I had an attack of blood poisoning." While on extended sick leave, he was advised to forego life in the smoky industrial Midlands; it was suggested that he try Canada or New Zealand.

Underhill read an advertisement in the *British Medical Journal* detailing a medical practice for sale in Mission, B.C., a small settlement on North America's faraway Pacific Coast, which was becoming more and more popular for British immigration. The description of the lush Fraser River valley, the clean air and the outdoor lifestyle, appealed to a man trying to regain his health, and it was not long before Underhill finalized the purchase of Dr. Boddington's Mission residence and medical practice. In 1884, Fred and Beatrice, with six children under the age of eight, set out to begin a new, challenging, and rewarding life in Canada.

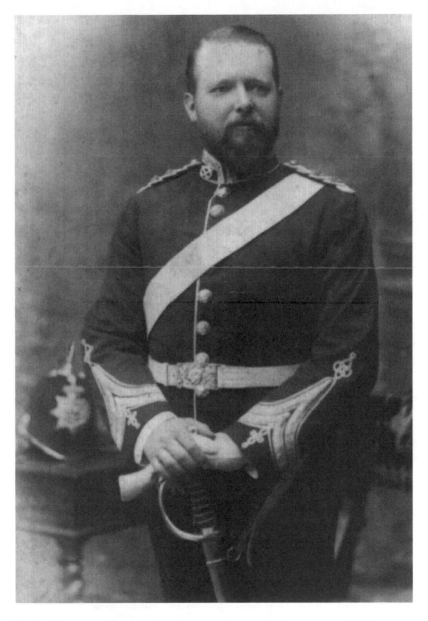

Before he came to Canada, Dr. Frederick Underhill was a surgeon in the volunteer battalion of the Fourth South Staffordshire Rifles.

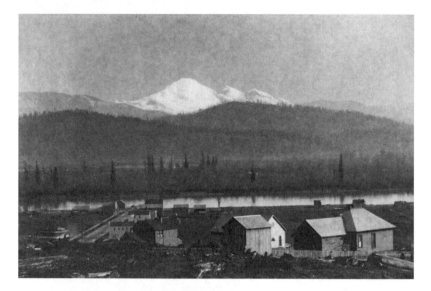

This is Mission, B.C., as it looked when the Underhills arrived here from England, having travelled with their six children across the Atlantic and then across Canada by train. They took up residence in one of these houses. Mount Baker can be seen in the distance.

They were accompanied by one of Beatrice's sisters, who helped look after the children, and a groom to care for the horses the doctor would need to make his rounds and which the family would use for transportation. Some years later he wrote: "I admit I was as green as grass as the average Englishman who comes out and I fell before that glowing advertisement without the faintest idea of what I was coming to, and bought the late Dr. Boddington's practice." Beatrice's sister remained with the family until she married an artist, Thomas Fripp, and went to live in Hatzic, another small community in the Fraser Valley.

Within days of their arrival in rural B.C., the doctor and his family experienced their first Canadian adventure. He recalled:

> I had been a few days in Dr. Boddington's house when a Mission neighbour came to me and said, 'I think you had better move your family out, as the flood is rising rapidly.' This was lively intelligence. I

at once put my wife and children—I had six then, under eight years of age—into a hay-wagon, and sent them to a place of safety. I stayed in the house thinking matters were not serious, but the next morning I had to leave by boat. We all landed in an old shack into every room of which the rain found admission and which was infested with rats. There we stayed, however, until this record flood subsided.

The family's first home in Canada was on the main street in Mission, the surgery located at ground level, and the living quarters upstairs.

Fred Underhill adapted quickly to his new life in the outdoors. He frequently took long horseback rides along deserted country roads through valley forests to see patients. Dr. Fred became a familiar figure in the area, always recognizable because of his neatly trimmed beard and his dapper appearance, enhanced by the elegant winged collar and carefully knotted tie he nearly always wore. It was said he only slightly demurred to the suggestion that he bore a resemblance to King Edward VII.

Successfully established in Mission, Dr. Underhill decided to build a new home that would more adequately accommodate his growing family. He chose a site on an acreage just outside the community. There he built a large home, again with a surgery on the main floor and, this time, with a stable built on the grounds to accommodate his horses.

It was an adventurous time for Underhill and his family. One winter he was thrown from his horse and fell heavily to the icy ground, hitting his head. When he regained consciousness, he was fortunate to find his animal had not strayed but had stood patiently nearby. Although shaken, Underhill remounted and continued his journey.

On another occasion, he was called urgently to Nicomen Island in the Fraser River. "The first day I got frozen in the ice of the Fraser and had to turn back. I had tried to row there in a dug-out. The second attempt was equally futile. My third attempt was on horseback and I landed through a snowdrift. I never got to my patient, who fortunately was not seriously ill and recovered."

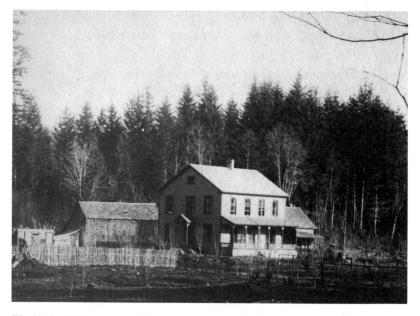

The Underhills' second residence was just outside of town and built to specifications set out by Dr. Fred. It included a surgery on the main floor and a stable to house several horses. The house unfortunately burned to the ground only a few years after it was completed.

In 1896, because there was a shortage of medical practitioners, the doctor was asked by the provincial government to undertake the treatment of some miners working in the interior Cariboo region, hundreds of miles from Mission. He welcomed the challenge with enthusiasm and over the next year made a number of long, arduous trips to isolated gold-mining camps.

On one occasion he was in Yale, in the Fraser Canyon, when he was asked to travel to Clinton to investigate the death of a Chinese man because the coroner and an inquest jury had markedly differing views on the cause of death. Underhill travelled by coach over Pavilion Mountain on what he described as "a magnificent journey." Upon arrival he found that the man had been buried beside a narrow, winding track about 200 feet above the river. In his report, Underhill wrote: "When we hoisted the coffin out, there was not much room to do anything. The coroner, Dr. Samson, sat on one side and I on the other, one leg in the grave and one dangling over the river. We had no instruments with us—when I left I was not entirely sure what I was to do—and had to make the post mortem with a Spanish clasp knife we had borrowed." His findings supported Samson's view.

Back in Mission, lively Beatrice Underhill's caregiving skills were soon nearly as respected as her husband's. When the doctor was away she often attended to minor complaints from regular patients and became expert at treating the steady stream of toothache sufferers who came to the door. Her self-taught dentistry was a no-anaesthetic-and-pliers approach. She cheerfully yanked teeth when the need was obvious, and patients always appreciated her post-operative treatment—a stiff belt of whiskey.

Although the mother of so many children, Beatrice still found time to be the organist at a small Anglican church in Mission. One daughter later recalled that her father was one of a handful who raised money to build the church, which was visited monthly by a travelling clergyman.

While attending to the miners in the Interior, Underhill took on other medical duties that cropped up in the sparsely populated central region of the province. He delivered the first white baby in the district of Horsefly, making a 70-mile detour on horseback to get there because of a raging forest fire.

The family then suffered a severe misfortune. While he was visiting one of the mining camps, Underhill received a telegram brought in on a horse-drawn freight wagon. It was many days old and contained fearful news. His new home in Mission had burned to the ground. The wire neglected to say if any of the family had succumbed or suffered injury. Worried and wanting to reach his family as soon as possible, Underhill took the first available transportation, a coach carrying $30,000 in gold with armed mounted guards at front and rear. It was heading for 150 Mile House, where Underhill hoped to send a cable to Mission to find out how his family had fared.

About 20 miles into the trip, the stage rolled while taking a sharp curve, and the driver was injured. Underhill treated the man while others righted the coach. One of the outriders took over driving the team of horses, and the doctor put on a gun and took up the guard's position. As it turned out, the wireless line at 150 Mile House was down. Not until the coach reached Ashcroft was Underhill able to

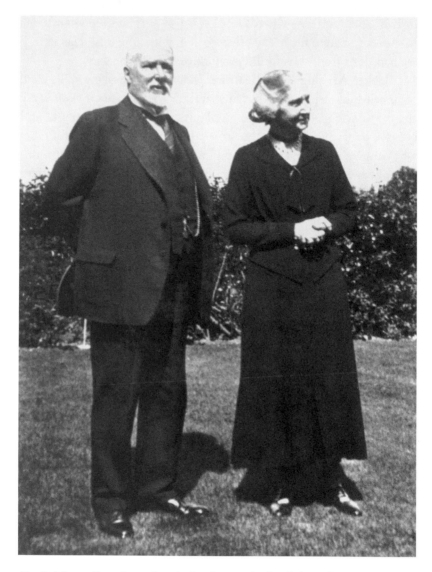

Frederick met Beatrice, a doctor's daughter, in his birthplace of Tipton, Staffordshire. In 1894, with six children under the age of eight, they moved to Canada. Both were involved first in the small community of Mission and later in the growing city of Vancouver.

discover that his family had escaped the fire and was safe and living in a rented New Westminster house.

With his home and office destroyed, Fred Underhill made some major decisions that affected the rest of his life. He decided in 1897 to return to Edinburgh for a year in order to study public-health administration, a field in which he had become keenly interested. While he was away, his wife supervised the building of a new home in Vancouver. The city was growing fast and offered more patients and better hospital facilities than were available in Mission. Underhill knew a practice in the city's affluent West End would do well and chose its residential heart, a district of quiet, tree-lined streets in a community that was growing at a steady rate.

For their new home, the Underhills picked a quiet spot on Barclay Street, overlooking English Bay beach. When the family moved into it nearly a year later, the children dubbed their home "The City Jail" because of the bars across the upstairs windows—Dr. Fred had had them installed to ensure that the children couldn't fall from the windows. As the children of a prominent, respected professional man, they lived the good life of an upper-middle-class family in a city that was only 15 years old when they took up residence there. The tempo of their life matched the clip-clop of horse-drawn vehicles, occasionally interrupted by the new "horseless carriage." A large veranda encircled the house, which sat amidst spacious gardens. There were only five other homes between theirs and the water.

Seven of the 13 Underhill children were born in Canada. The first six were born in Tipton: Muriel Beatrice, the eldest, born in 1886, followed by Reginald, Ella Margaretta, Frederic Clare, James Theodore, and Charles Bertram. Born after them, in Canada, were William Leslie Lamb, Sybil Mary, Enid Anna Kathleen, Helen Elizabeth, John Edward, Benjamin Arthur (who died before his second birthday), and Richard Walter, born in 1907. It was a large, lively group of children, well known wherever the family lived.

Mealtimes at the Underhills were times for voicing opinions, although the manners and mores of the Edwardian age were still observed. Dr. Underhill, who had many outside responsibilities and interests, was not a strict disciplinarian, but watched his offspring with an often-bemused affection. His wife was the family spark

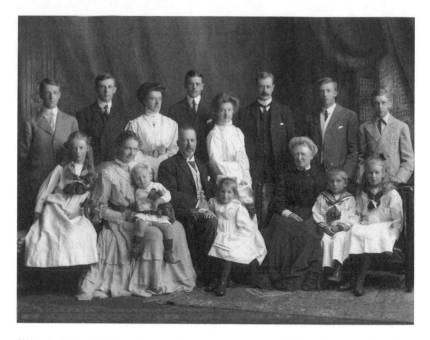

This Underhill family photograph was taken prior to 1914 when the older boys departed for the war in Europe. The picture includes everyone except Benjamin, who died before the age of two. The older two sons, Reginald and Charles, were killed during World War I in France. Pictured (left to right) are: (back row) Charles, Clare, Ella, Reginald, Muriel and her husband, Dr. Harold Dyer, Jim, and Bill; (front row) Sybil, Mrs. Underhill holding Dick, Dr. Underhill, Helen, Aunt Mina, Jack, and Enid.

plug, a lively, fun-loving mother who took an interest in the many involvements of her brood. The house was a warm jumble of piano music, tennis racquets, and croquet mallets. Friends were always welcome and the place usually swarmed with them.

On many a soft, lemonade-sipping summer night, the trill of the birds was accompanied by a chorus of voices from the porch, rendering the latest songs. Some must have seemed a trifle risqué to the doctor; these were the opening years of the 20th century, a fresh age when hearts were young and gay. None of them could have dreamed of the tragedies that lay ahead, for during the years leading up to 1914, Vancouver was filled with wild hopes and dreams. It was a golden time for the Underhills and all those like them.

City's first health officer

Dr. Underhill had become one of the few local doctors with special qualifications in public health; it was not long before he was asked to become bacteriologist for the city, an unpaid position. He undertook the work with interest and, in a less-than-spotless community, became a strong advocate for sanitation and for public education in personal hygiene and preventive medicine.

His medical practice flourished in the West End, where he became a well-known and respected member of the growing city. His reports as bacteriologist engendered considerable debate at meetings of the Health Committee and Vancouver City Council. His views, expressed forcefully and sincerely, soon became well known, and his opinions on local health issues were frequently sought.

In 1904 the chairman of the health committee, Dr. W.D. Brydone-Jack, asked Underhill to give up his practice and become the city's first full-time, paid medical health officer. It was the beginning of a long, colourful career filled with its share of controversy, crisis, and outstanding accomplishment. "I was always fond of public health work and though it meant giving up a lucrative practice, I could not resist the temptation," Underhill commented. "When I undertook this I admit I had hopes of some provincial or dominion appointment, for I saw the necessity at that time for such an appointment, but it did not come."

From the day he took on the job until the epidemic of 1918, Underhill watched Vancouver grow from a city of 40,000 people to one of 110,000. It was a city in which he played an essential and dedicated role. In the beginning, his staff consisted of only three people—a sanitary inspector and two plumbing inspectors—but in later years his support staff numbered in the 20s. Not surprising, considering that during his career Underhill fulfilled the functions of police surgeon, city bacteriologist, and analyst.

Ever curious and anxious for answers, Underhill happily delved into new problems and the mysteries of disease and treatment as he found them. The people of Vancouver quickly learned that he wouldn't prescribe a new treatment for them that he wouldn't give to his own children. Sometimes he would even try out vaccines and medicines on his brood before using them on the general public. One son complained that he lived with a constantly sore arm. His sons and daughters also recalled being asked to help with his projects. On one occasion this entailed going to the waterfront to check that the devices meant to prevent rats from climbing along the mooring lines of ships in port were securely in place. This was during a period when Underhill was intent on establishing and policing every imaginable safeguard against a possible outbreak of bubonic plague.

One of Underhill's earliest and most difficult tasks as medical health officer was escorting lepers to D'Arcy Island in the Strait of Georgia. He said the inhabitants appeared to be Orientals or Native people and observed, "A very bad situation used to prevail upon this island." The government in Victoria ran the installation, and new patients identified for exile from Vancouver travelled first to Esquimalt, and from there were transported to the island. Underhill expressed his deep concerns to his wife and admitted that each trip to this tragic, barren island left him emotionally drained: "In those days of which I speak, we had to hire a tug, erect a tent at the back of the tug and take these cases to D'Arcy Island. As a rule no one was anxious to take the job on. They were shipped to the island, provisions and water were conveyed to them from time to time and they used to hoist a flag when they were in distress. It was a very unsatisfactory state of affairs."

Many of Underhill's new ideas for Vancouver were costly and not always appreciated by taxpayers, city fathers, and merchants, but he was adamant in his beliefs, never swerving if he believed he was right. His first crusade was cleaning up the city by organizing the first real garbage collection. He stalked city streets to ensure that manure piles were removed regularly. Always well dressed from his hat to his shining boots, he carefully picked his way through the odoriferous piles of assorted garbage that littered the streets and alleys, seeing them as a constant menace to health.

He also encouraged vaccinations against smallpox and various measures to control other infectious diseases. There were loud complaints when he insisted on regulations to ensure cleanliness of food handlers and restaurant kitchens. Water was another of his concerns. Always fearful of an outbreak of typhoid, Underhill was well aware that people in outlying districts still drank well water, which easily became contaminated by farm animals and outhouses. He wanted to ensure that as many people as possible in Vancouver and the surrounding region had access to clean water.

Vancouver waterworks

As a result, Underhill became an advocate for the immediate expansion of Vancouver's drinking-water supply system. By 1889, the Vancouver Water Works Company had completed a water line from the Capilano River, across First Narrows, to a reservoir in Stanley Park. The city purchased the company in 1891, and for 17 years this was Vancouver's sole water source. It was, however, subject to disruption, as ships entering the Narrows at low tide often broke the pipe with their keels, and it could be days before the pipe was repaired. Distribution to homes in the city was not often disrupted, but low levels of water in the reservoir were often a concern.

Underhill was quick to point out that the system was inadequate for the growing city, and before long councillors approved a water-system upgrade. Building began in 1906 and ended in 1910. It involved constructing a new wood stave and cast-iron pipeline running from Seymour Creek on the North Shore down the mountain, through a submerged main across Burrard Inlet, and then into the city. By 1911 the Little Mountain Reservoir had been completed to augment the distribution system, which was centred at Georgia and Chilco streets. The new system cost $300,000 and was financed by water rates charged to homeowners and businesses.

Underhill became a familiar figure to homesteaders in North Vancouver as he tramped over trails, through forests and up into the mountains to check the purity of Vancouver's water supply. Sometimes group photos were taken during waterworks inspections, and, as always, even among 50-odd people the doctor was easily identifiable because he was the only one sporting a winged collar and tie. Dr. Henry Young, the provincial medical officer and another keen advocate of preventive medicine and clean water, often accompanied Underhill on these excursions. As time went by, Underhill was able to make part of the trip in the city's solid-tire Stanley Steamer automobile, which wheezed its way up the rough roads built in the early part of the century.

In 1910 Underhill was confronted by the outbreak of typhoid he had feared. The number of cases quickly climbed to 265, but it would undoubtedly have been far worse without the abundance of clean, pure water now available to the young city. The always-progressive doctor had an often-expounded credo by which he lived. He told the city fathers: "You can never be satisfied with conditions as they are."

Crime detection

Underhill's offices were in the building that housed the city hall and the jail on Powell Street. His laboratory was on the top floor. Shortly into his tenure he hired an assistant, a man named John Fleming Cullen Brown Vance who had particular expertise in chemistry and metallurgy and took over operation of the lab.

Vance soon was appointed city analyst and, eventually, assistant medical health officer. He and Underhill worked closely together, becoming lifelong friends. Vance's knowledge of minerals and chemicals resulted in the conviction of a number of prominent criminals of this era; one reporter dubbed Vance "Canada's Sherlock Holmes." He worked closely with the police department on several criminal cases and within a few years was given the honorary title of detective inspector. Before Vance retired in 1946, the laboratory was second to none. He had a staff of 17 working for the city, the province, and, on occasion, for the federal government, providing scientific information that often sent criminals to jail or, now and then, cleared the accused.

Frequently, Underhill and Vance went together on tours of inspection through the crowded downtown sections of Vancouver and its teeming, always-busy Chinatown. They learned that the Chinese had developed a system of underground passages to offer protection should there be riots or outside hostility. So that the tunnels could be included in health inspections, Underhill and Vance spent time learning where they were located.

Vancouver at this time was made up primarily of immigrants from Great Britain, but Underhill also had a variety of experiences among the city's small ethnic communities. His care to include

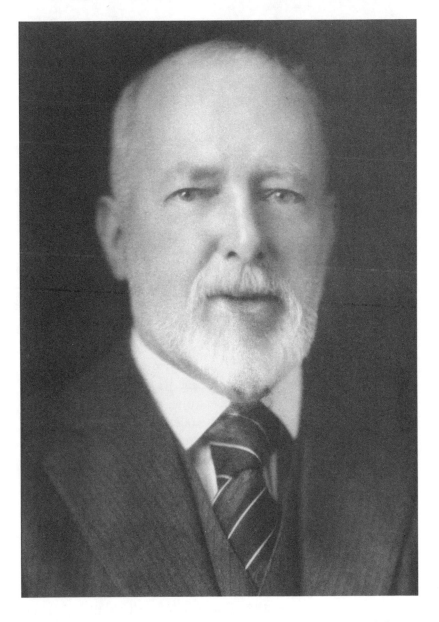

Dr. Frederick Theodore Underhill had firm convictions. He maintained that "you can never be satisfied with conditions as they are." He only slightly demurred when it was suggested that he resembled King Edward VII.

them in public health was unusual, even if many of his attitudes were typical of the time. He said the Hindus, because of their caste system, had given him "no end of trouble," but said, "I must confess to a liking for the Chinaman. If you are absolutely straight with him and make him understand what you want, he will do what you want. But if he can do you up in a knot he will, he enjoys it." He said he had little trouble with the Japanese.

Underhill's beliefs and recommendations were often disputed by those who thought the measures he advocated were costly and unnecessary. He sometimes rubbed city fathers the wrong way—and a few misguided colleagues tried to paint him as a carbolic-soap handwashing fussbudget from old England—but he was steadfast and insistent. In an age when cleanliness mattered less, he was a zealous advocate of handwashing. Friends described him as a modern man with a good sense of humour who didn't hanker for the good old days, but looked to the future.

Underhill was always a busy man, sponsoring a whole range of initiatives on top of his day-to-day work. His views and practices in the field of public health helped reduce Vancouver's infant mortality rate to one of the lowest in North America. He established a day nursery and an employment bureau for working mothers and their children, and he was one of the founders of an early Vancouver organization known as the Associated Charities, a forerunner of the United Way. He was also responsible for the city's relief department.

Despite these charitable concerns, Underhill had little time for malingerers and those who refused to help themselves. His tough, no-nonsense side showed through when a group of transients raised a ruckus at city hall, demanding relief. The paper described the transients as mostly men from the old country who had only been in town a short time. Underhill went to the old city hall, where arrangements had been made to house 100 of them temporarily, but bristled and became outraged when he was told that some of the men had refused jobs clearing lots at $2 per day. It was not an insignificant sum at the time. He gave them a "right from the shoulder" dressing-down, telling them that while the city was prepared to help, they also had to be prepared to help themselves. He noted with disgust that seven of them had appeared in court earlier in the day on charges of being drunk. They learned quickly that he was no soft touch.

Most important, Underhill was a pioneer in the control of infectious diseases. With regard to these responsibilities, he commented: "The next important thing I found vital was to be in absolute control of the infectious diseases in the city by insisting all medical men and all schools report such diseases. Now I think I can safely assert there is not a city where the system is more thorough." He introduced quarantine signs for the windows of homes stricken by diphtheria, scarlet fever, or other contagious diseases in order to warn others to stay away. Such signs would proliferate during the visit of the Spanish Lady.

THE SPANISH LADY ARRIVES

The first outbreak of the flu in North America occurred late in February 1918 at a military camp in Kansas. An army private reported ill with the flu one day, and by that evening there were 100 cases. By week's end, there were 500. It was confined to the base for a couple of weeks, but the number of cases escalated quickly, and by March 11 the outbreak was no longer contained.

It was not long before officials in Philadelphia also issued a bulletin informing residents that the Spanish influenza had arrived. Boston, however, was the first large U.S. city to report a major epidemic and a large number of cases. Sixty sailors were sick aboard a medical receiving ship at Commonwealth Pier there, and more were being admitted to Chelsea Naval Hospital. Within three weeks of the flu's arrival, the military base at Camp Devens, near Boston, reported that it was losing 100 young men a day. Boston eventually had more cases and more deaths than most other U.S. cities.

Exactly how and when the Spanish Lady first set foot in Canada is unclear, but the pandemic was well underway in Europe when the ship *Araguaya* left England on June 26. She arrived in Canada in early July, with 175 cases of flu among the 763 soldiers aboard. There were also sailors who contracted the disease while bringing home their countrymen. One young Canadian doctor, H.H. Geggie, was among the first to notice the large influx of sick men arriving at St. Jean, Quebec. It took several calls to Montreal, each one to a more senior official, before he was able to convince the military that the

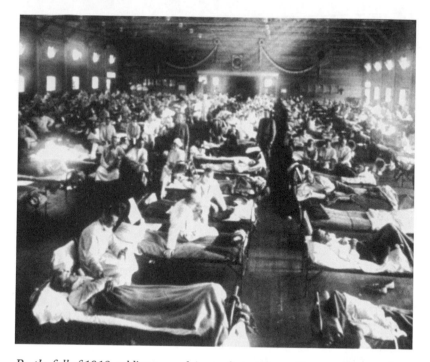

By the fall of 1918, soldiers were dying so fast at Camp Funston, Kansas, that corpses had to be piled up like cords of wood outside until coffins could be found for them. Pictured here is the emergency hospital at Camp Funston at the height of the epidemic.

crisis they had discussed in March had arrived. It took many more calls and pleas to Ottawa before he received extra medical help.

The fact that initially all the sick soldiers were treated at Quebec army hospitals kept the Spanish Lady isolated for only a short time. As the flu spread, it began to affect replacement soldiers going overseas. Recruits embarked from Quebec City or Montreal, the same centres where returning veterans were being hospitalized. Flu deaths became common at sea on the voyage to Europe as well as on the return. The troopship *City of Cairo* sailed from Quebec on September 28 and arrived at Devonport, England, on October 11. She left with 1,057 soldiers aboard; nearly all became ill. Thirty-five were buried at sea. The *Hunstead* sailed from Montreal on October 4. Thirty-nine of the 1,549 soldiers who embarked died during the voyage, and 73 were immediately transferred to hospital upon arriving in England. The *Victoria*, which sailed from Quebec on October 6 with 1,230 aboard, buried 28 at sea and had a peak of 307 men sick during the crossing.

Quebec hit hard

Before long, the situation in Montreal was appalling, particularly in areas where families lived in close proximity in rooming houses and tenements. The number of new cases soared, and there were many fatalities. Funeral processions plugged downtown streets, while undertakers and gravediggers couldn't keep up with the demand for their services. Frequently funerals were held for several members of a family at one time.

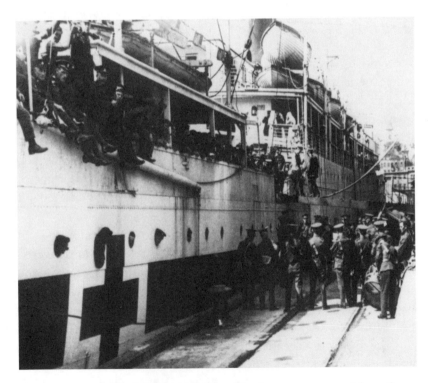

The pandemic was well underway in Europe when troops returned from the front, unknowingly bringing the virus home with them. Pictured here are veterans unloading from a hospital ship in Halifax, Nova Scotia.

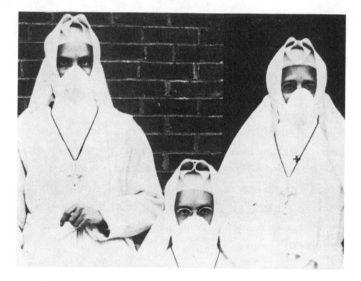

Nuns cared for flu victims in 1918 in hard-hit Quebec, which lost 13,000 people to the flu by the end of 1919.

One story, just one among hundreds, concerned Arthur Lapointe, who experienced a devastating homecoming for a war-weary soldier. He had contracted flu in France and had had a recurrence at a camp in England before heading home. Upon arriving in Montreal, he learned that he had lost three brothers and two sisters to the flu; all of them had died within a nine-day period. Roman Catholic orphanages in the province were reporting a record number of children available for adoption as the Spanish Lady carried off fathers and mothers.

Quebec residents found themselves commandeered for unusual duties. In Montreal, it was the police and firemen who delivered food and fuel to families in need. In other communities, women's service groups or churches organized volunteers. Schools closed and teachers volunteered to work in hospitals or mustered older students to fill in where they were needed.

The most seriously affected province was undoubtedly Quebec. It was the first to be struck with the flu, and no preparations had been made to fight it outside of the military. The picture was not much better across the country, but officials in other locations had more time to prepare. Quebec provincial and municipal health officials took charge in most cases, recommending bed rest and particular attention to personal hygiene. Nothing else was available. The better-prepared Canadian military did offer some relief. Although hard pressed like medical services everywhere, it sent help from Montreal to the small Quebec lumber town of Shawinigan, where 200 plant employees were ill.

The most pressing problem was finding or creating venues for isolation hospitals so that those who were ill could be removed to them and kept away from the general population. Emergency space was at a premium, and administrators began requisitioning hotels, dormitories, schools, and any appropriate building that could serve as an isolation hospital. Meanwhile, by October 13 public worship in devout Montreal was suspended.

Travelling east and west

While soldiers had been hospitalized in Quebec since June, there were few signs of the advance of the disease in the rest of the country at first. It wasn't until August that its presence became evident in Toronto and parts of Ontario, particularly in communities near military hospitals. Then, seemingly overnight, there were cases everywhere.

It was the troops coming home that spread the disease so fast. One Canadian Pacific Railway conductor prided himself on having dropped off returning soldiers at all the major cities and at many of the small towns in each province as his train wound its way through the Maritimes, Ontario, and the Prairies to Vancouver. Rail travel was the engine that led the Spanish Lady on her trek across the vast interior reaches and the mountains to the sea. During their days-long journeys, even healthy military personnel were often taken ill, some of them dying en route, while other soldiers, seemingly on the mend, took the disease home with them. There was a sad irony to it all. These men, who had volunteered to fight and risk their lives for Canada and their loved ones, had survived, but now they were unwittingly bringing sickness and death home with them.

It was some time before authorities realized the pandemic was spreading along the country's rail routes. The failure to restrict train travel early on was one of the terrible oversights made in fighting the Spanish Lady in Canada. It was too late when, in November, the CPR reported that 40 to 45 towns had quarantined themselves and would be closed to trains. Eventually rail traffic was curtailed almost completely, but not before thousands of passengers and employees had been taken ill and travel had dropped off severely because of the number of people stricken by the flu.

The disease travelled both east and west from Quebec. By early September the Spanish Lady had moved into New Brunswick, although no one knows how hard it was hit. According to provincial epidemiologist Dr. Christofer Balram, information about the number of deaths in New Brunswick does not exist, an indication that record-keeping was not a priority in 1918. A figure of 1,400 is plausible, based on the average death toll in other provinces of one percent of the population.

From there the disease moved into all of the Maritimes. There had been five deaths in Sydney, Nova Scotia, by the end of the September, and the caseload was rising in Halifax. Prince Edward Island set up a ferry passenger inspection in an effort to keep the flu out, but the Spanish Lady came anyway. The island's statistics for 1918 and 1919 record almost 400 deaths from flu and pneumonia, despite the editorial opinions of the local newspaper. *The Guardian* took a hard line, contending that the outbreak was a case of mind over matter. It argued that fear and not flu was the real enemy, declaring: "Remove fear and Spanish influenza will vanish as quickly as she came." Newfoundland, not part of Canada in 1918, was also being ravaged, particularly the native communities along the Labrador coast.

Ontario succumbs

On October 5 the Toronto *Globe and Mail* ran the headline "Spanish Flu Spreading" and reported that "the disease has a firm hold in other municipalities and there have been 500 to 600 cases in Toronto with nine deaths." In the same edition it was reported that two doctors and 12 nurses had been sent to the community of Renfrew to "check the spread of the disease."

Within days the Almonte Hospital was overflowing with 100 cases, while Georgetown Hospital had 50 patients and had seen the death of its first medical man, Dr. James Richard Nixon. One Ottawa hospital reported 18 nurses off sick, and Kitchener recorded its first death. There were 400 reported flu cases in Port Hope.

The disease became unstoppable. Forty died in London, Ontario, and it was estimated that there were at least 1,000 cases in the area. Toronto officials announced that no one with a cough or cold should leave their dwelling and discussed imposing penalties on anyone caught on the street with a cough or without a handkerchief. The saddest story of the day concerned a man named John Lewis; all the members of his large family had died of the flu. He was the last to be stricken, and he too died.

Making matters more difficult was the death toll among medical men. Reported to have reached 200 across the country, it compounded the problem of tending to the needs of the ever-increasing number of patients. As the flu spread, so did fear of the unknown; despite this, doctors, nurses, and hospital staff often displayed great courage and devotion. Already short-handed because so many professionals were serving overseas, they worked long hours with few breaks and little sleep. During the pandemic many, many health-care workers paid with their lives.

As the shortage of hospital beds, doctors, and nurses became more acute, one caregiver decided to take an unusual step. Dr. Margaret Patterson knew something must be done to save the lives of the sick and dying, so she instituted a training program for volunteers that was described as a course in general preparation for nursing at home. Sponsored by the Ontario Emergency Volunteer Health Authority, the courses began October 16 and were held initially in the Parliament buildings. She told her first students: "We must band together to fight this disease which seems to affect chiefly the respiratory organs and we are very much concerned with the heart's action." Graduates of the intensive two-day course were known as Sisters of Service (SOS), and each received a badge upon graduating. Patterson's programs proved effective in training hundreds of women in the best methods for reducing lung congestion and keeping fevers down, as well as for treating patients in the home. In fact, the program was so effective that it was soon taken up in other parts of the city and in other communities across Ontario.

In Kingston a group of SOS women organized nursing quarters in the Great War Veterans and Army and Navy Veterans buildings, and these became emergency isolation hospitals. In Chatham there were 40 to 50 flu cases by October 21, and the Volunteer Health Auxiliary introduced an SOS training program. Still the death toll mounted. In Guelph there were 10 deaths in 24 hours, and in Windsor there were 15 new cases and 5 deaths in a similar period.

In Ottawa, the health board asked businesses to close at 4 p.m. and offices at 3 p.m. in order to reduce the amount of time people would be together and the disease could be transmitted. The same kind of futile gesture was made in other places across the country. Ottawa lost 500 residents to the flu, a large proportion of them living in the crowded area of Lowertown just east of the Parliament Buildings.

At the height of the epidemic on October 16, an irate mayor, Harold Fisher, stated: "People died last night because they had nobody to look after them last week when they had nothing but a mild attack of influenza. People will also die next week unless they have someone to take care of them tonight." That night there were 900 people in hospital with the flu in Ottawa.

The outbreak in Ontario was intense, but briefer than in some other parts of the country. As suddenly as she arrived, the Spanish Lady began to take her leave; by November 1, *The Globe and Mail* was able to announce a marked improvement except in the western half of the province. Bans on public meetings were lifted. Ottawa cautiously announced that it would reopen churches on November 11, and Kingston closed its emergency hospital at the Army and Navy building. The people of Kitchener, reported to have greatly missed the comfort of the church bells pealing, could be happy again as their churches reopened.

Flu reaches Manitoba

In 1918, Winnipeg, Manitoba, was the third-largest city in Canada and took a great deal of pride in its position of prestige. It had a better medical infrastructure than other prairie cities, allowing Medical Health Officer Dr. Alex. J. Douglas to warn the city's 260,000 people on September 25 that the flu was "coming for sure." The first victims had been two soldiers among 20 sick men taken from a westbound train two weeks before. Up till then, Winnipeggers read of the dreaded flu striking Saskatchewan and B.C. before they knew of any local deaths.

How Winnipeg was able to hold the Spanish Lady at arm's length for so long is not clear. Dr. Douglas, like other health officials, was aware of the need to allay people's fears, and he may have delayed confirming cases. Doctors in Winnipeg did their best to prevent panic and frequently reiterated that the situation was better in Manitoba than elsewhere, giving credit to the early closure of public places. Perhaps it was simply that family doctors did not always report cases of flu to the health department.

The city's mayor and council decided early on that quarantine and closure would be the route to take and closed Winnipeg's schools and places of entertainment. Despite this, by October 14 there were 80 reported cases in the province as a whole and the number had doubled to more than 160 by the following day.

By October 17, Manitoba authorities were boarding all westbound trains before they entered the province, stopping them at Rainy River and Kenora in an attempt to get those who were ill into quarantine as quickly as possible. Small towns along the rail line began to refuse people entry as the death rate climbed. In Riverton, stores were ordered to open for only three hours a day and to serve no more than two customers at a time.

Two among the dead were William Code, aged 78, whose only son had died in the Riel Rebellion, and a young nurse, a recent arrival from Galt, Ontario, whose name was listed in the *Winnipeg Free Press* only as Nurse Studeman. There was sadness when people read about Alan McLeod, a young flyer who had distinguished himself over France by shooting down three of eight attacking enemy aircraft. He survived the dogfight, crashing his riddled plane into no man's land, and was awarded the Victoria Cross for gallantry, only to die of the flu six months later in Canada.

Winnipeg officials quarantined all homes in which people were down with the flu and urged everyone to practise careful personal hygiene—in particular, to wash their hands as often as possible. There was a $50 fine for spitting in public. Dr. William Boyd of Manitoba's

Medical College made a trip to the famous Mayo Clinic in Rochester, Minnesota, to obtain a vaccine for use against the flu. Newspaper stories were not enthusiastic about the effectiveness of the vaccine and quoted numerous doctors, including B.C.'s Dr. Young, as saying it was of questionable value. Meanwhile, the *Winnipeg Free Press* was advertising a medicine for the sick called "Mathieu's Spirits." It was undoubtedly one of the worst concoctions created during the pandemic. Containing a mixture of spirit of tar and cod liver oil, a large bottle sold for 35 cents.

Winnipeg continued to downplay the severity of the outbreak, a seemingly unusual view in light of the circumstances. The *Winnipeg Free Press* reported that while the flu was "spreading rapidly," medical officials maintained that Winnipeg was not doing badly in comparison with other cities, even though this was no longer true. School cafeterias prepared food for families too sick to make their own meals; it was discovered that everyone in one family of nine was in bed, too sick to get up. Within days there was sharp criticism of the decision to provide food to the sick because of the effect it would have on the city's image. One newspaper said Winnipeg was "looking like London in the plague rather than a western city in the twentieth century." Winnipeg prided itself on being modern and progressive, and the sight of pestilence in the streets, even if conditions were the same everywhere else, did not appeal to the city fathers.

An enterprising *Free Press* reporter described one unusual event resulting from the flu pandemic. Harry Fleckman and Dora Wiseman were to be married, but instead of the usual joyous affair, their families decided on a "sacrificial wedding," a ceremony resurrected from ancient Jewish folklore and described as a ceremony similar to an exorcism. Hundreds attended the 3 p.m. rites at the local Jewish cemetery, led by rabbis Khanovitch and Gorodsky. A Jewish band played "weird and mystical music and an elderly gentleman delivered a passionate address. This was followed by much moaning and crying before the hat was passed for the usual donation for the married couple." The reporter noted, "It was a strange custom revived from the past of an ancient race."

By mid-October, evening temperatures were dipping below freezing, and Dr. Douglas made a desperate appeal for volunteers to assist nurses and to help with food deliveries, although 10,000 meals had been served already. As prairie temperatures dropped lower, nobody sick with the flu dared venture outside the house for anything, so those who were not sick performed an extra service in all these frigid communities. The hard-hit city of Brandon announced that only people without kitchens, such as roomers who were not boarders, would be allowed to eat in restaurants.

The epidemic in Winnipeg reached and passed its zenith around November 20; by then 4,400 people had been released from quarantine and there was room available in some hospitals that had been "taxed to the limit for three weeks." While the number of new cases rose and fell erratically, the general trend was now downward, and public schools and buildings were reopened.

Into Saskatchewan and Alberta

The first recorded death from the flu in Saskatchewan, which had a population of about 725,000, was in Regina. The city was already trying to deal with an outbreak of smallpox. The death of a man named Robert Callander was noted with gloom by Regina's medical health officer, Dr. M.R. Bow. He told his city's 30,000 people: "We are liable to have trouble ... it is sweeping the country and we can't be immune." Dr. Bow's words were prophetic personally as well as publicly; it was not long before he was stricken.

Regina opened an emergency isolation unit, and provincial health officer Dr. M.M. Seymour stated there would be severe penalties if new cases were not reported promptly. As the Spanish Lady took hold, hospitals filled quickly, and by October 15 there were seven people dead. One of these was a pioneer priest, Father A. Suffa of St. Mary's Church, who had arrived in the area in 1903, two years before Saskatchewan became a province.

Unlike many other communities, Regina did not close its public schools until officials found that frightened parents were keeping their children at home anyway, and classes were nearly empty.

Smaller communities like Assiniboia and Estevan were particularly hard hit when the few doctors they shared became exhausted by the long hours and the difficulties of frigid prairie travel.

The Regina Ministerial Association felt the need to send a message to parishioners when there were 1,500 reported cases of flu, 500 of them very severe. Unable to address their congregations in person because of church closures, the ministerial association message appeared on the front page of *The Leader-Post:* "You are living in trying times, but you must keep your faith in God."

Lieutenant-Governor Sir Charles Lake also issued a proclamation urging everyone to show a spirit of neighbourliness by calling on those living nearby to ensure "they are all right."

Mrs. Gladys Nelson from the small town of Outlook was one of many women who over the weeks cooked meals for those unable to feed themselves. She worked so hard that she was made an honorary member of the St. John Ambulance Society. Only three people died in tiny Outlook.

The annual report of the Bureau of Public Health states that Saskatchewan lost 3,906 people in 1918. Regina recorded 255 deaths and Saskatoon, with a population of about 24,000, recorded 200; the highest on a percentage basis was Moosejaw, with 166 victims, 7.6 percent per 1,000 of population. Saskatchewan later produced a breakdown of the occupations of victims: farmers, 1,189; housewives, 896; electricians, 5; merchants, 53; nurses, 17; students, 53; policemen, 8; schoolteachers, 31; and railway men, 63.

By the time the Spanish Lady reached Alberta, fear had taken possession of many public officials, and as a result some extreme measures were put in place. Calgary, a city of 72,000 people, and Edmonton, with approximately 66,000, were told by local newspapers that "the plague" had arrived. By the time the flu left, it had claimed more than 4,300 people out of a population of about 560,000.

The first suspected cases were again soldiers travelling by train, who in this case were taken to a Calgary hospital. Hundreds of soldiers were returning to the cities daily. Officials ordered that anyone travelling on public transport or appearing on the streets wear a mask. Spitting was prohibited and weddings were limited to 12 people. All schools and places of entertainment were shut down. Provincial authorities prepared signs in English and Russian, the province's two major languages, warning that the flu had arrived and proper precautions must be taken. A large number of Russian and

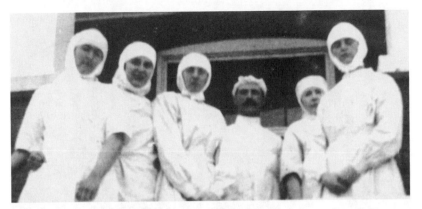

Teachers volunteered to help nurses battle the flu at an isolation hospital in Lloydminster, a centre straddling the Alberta–Saskatchewan border.

eastern European immigrants had chosen Alberta as their new home early in the century, and in 1918 many did not yet speak English.

Trying to take a light-hearted view of a death-dealing situation, *The Edmonton Journal* printed a poem entitled "The Flooies'll Get You."

> Once there was a businessman,
> Who would not wear a mask.
> He said it interfered with
> The performance of his task.
> He tried it for a minute—
> Then he promptly took it off,
> And now his staff is haunted by
> The memory of his cough.
> The Flooies sure will get you
> If you don't watch out.

Communities such as Lethbridge, Taber, and Pincher Creek ordered all CPR passenger cars sealed as they passed through; no one was permitted to disembark. Roadblocks were set up and manned by provincial police officers who forbade travellers from entering towns.

The coal town of Drumheller totted up an astounding 750 cases, severely affecting the production of coal, vital for the coming winter. The community sent out a desperate plea for medical help and

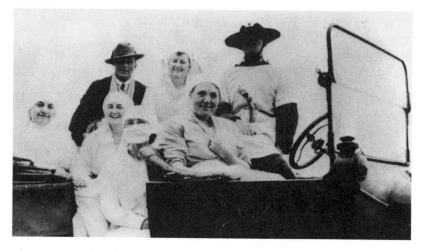

A group of workers from the emergency flu hospital in Milo, Alberta.

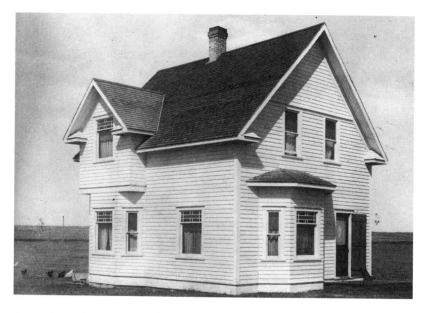

Throughout the country, buildings of all kinds were pressed into service as emergency hospitals.

managerial assistance, as most of the stricken mine managers were the people who ran the town.

Alberta's extreme regulations soon brought complaints from citizens about everything from the length of home quarantines to the fact that some neighbours were cheating by not reporting cases to authorities. Some doctors questioned the need for quarantine and were slow to fill out reports, which may have sparked even more complaints.

At least one doctor knew the value of seclusion. Charles Mitchel of Lethbridge realized that as a hard-pressed, overworked physician he was a prime target for the virus, as was his wife. In preparation for the inevitable, the couple stocked their home with fluids, moved their beds close to the fireplace, took to them the moment their temperatures rose, and stayed there until they recovered.

This province gave its name to another of the foul-smelling poultices found across the country. The directions for the Alberta Pack were:

> Peel 10 pounds of onions (for an adult), run them through a meat processor with the finest cutter available, put them in a dishpan, add about six or seven pounds of fine salt, stir together on the stove until it is too hot to hold in the hand, add enough flour to thicken so the juice will not run, wrap in oilcloth to keep the bedclothes clean, not to be worn for more than ten hours, remove and rub with soft towels and sweet oil and alcohol.

Other poultices called for potatoes, bran, lard mixed with camphor, chloroform, or a half-and-half mixture of lard and turpentine.

The pandemic had such an effect in Alberta that the key issues in a later Calgary election campaign were the flu, related health issues, and the city's ability to handle the situation.

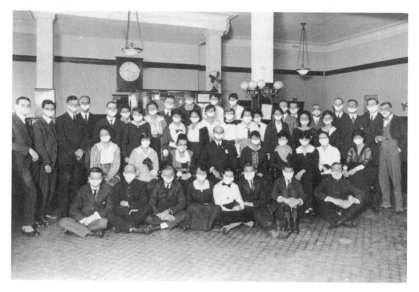

Staff at the Canadian Bank of Commerce in Calgary, Alberta, pose in protective masks in 1918.

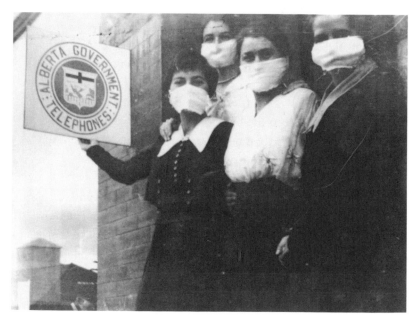

Telephone operators wearing masks in High River, Alberta, circa 1918–1919.

FLU STALKS VANCOUVER
AND VICTORIA

As the Spanish Lady continued her waltz westward, she was closely watched in B.C. by the three top medical men, who knew they would face a major challenge when she arrived on the Pacific coast: Dr. Underhill, Dr. Young, and Dr. Price. They kept in touch with each other and with public health officials across the country as the disease leapfrogged its way from one community to another, sometimes avoiding a city, a town, or village for a few days, but almost always returning to take its toll.

By September 1918 provincial and civic officials realized that the arrival of this terrible pandemic was imminent and unavoidable. Newspaper reports suggested that no matter how remote or seemingly isolated a town or village might be, or what precautions were taken, there was little defence against the flu. Physicians in both Vancouver and Victoria hoped fervently, although they knew it was almost impossible, that a cure or at least an effective treatment would be found before the pandemic reached the coast. Everyone watched and waited. Calmed to some extent by reassuring public statements from Dr. Underhill, who was making as many preparations as possible, Vancouver residents concentrated on their regular routines and tried not to worry.

They took some comfort in the underplayed stories typical of local news coverage. The press was the public's main source of information in 1918. Stories of the flu's toll in the east frequently underplayed the threat and even seemed quite sanguine about it. One report mentioned only the "discomfiting effects" of the disease. It isn't clear whether this coverage reflected a lack of appreciation of the flu's seriousness or whether the powers that were deliberately downplayed its severity. Vancouver readers were told correctly that precautions—not defined—were the best way to beat this new disease, but they were also told that the flu was a short-lived sickness, producing no permanent serious results, with the sufferer generally prostrate for only a few days, "during which he suffers the acme of discomfort." This description would in many cases prove to be far from the truth. October 1918 would be a month like no other in the short history of British Columbia. It would leave communities throughout the province reeling and its largest cities, Vancouver and Victoria, struggling to save lives.

As the Spanish Lady made her way to Vancouver in early October, Dr. Underhill and his wife were still quietly suffering their own deep personal loss: the death of their two oldest sons. Like many Canadian families, they had dreaded each day's news from the war front as casualties mounted in France. They had sent five sons off to war and now knew that Reginald and Charles would never return. They were dead in Flanders Fields. Five sisters mourned them, as well as the three brothers still serving overseas and the two boys who, too young to enlist, had remained at home.

The two oldest boys had enlisted at the outbreak of war and, as members of the Seventh Battalion Duke of Connaughts Own Rifles, went overseas in 1914 with the first Canadian contingent. Eager to see action, they then switched to the British army because they felt the Canadians would be deployed too late. Many people thought the war would be over within a year. Reginald joined the Middlesex Regiment and Charles was with the West Yorkshire Regiment. The war dragged on, and while Reginald and Charles both survived the slaughter at the battle of Mons, 1916 proved fatal for them. They were killed within eight months of each other and are buried in cemeteries only seven miles apart. It was a tragic blow for the family.

Even though well advanced in his career, Underhill at 60 was a man of prodigious energy and drive who never stopped working. He

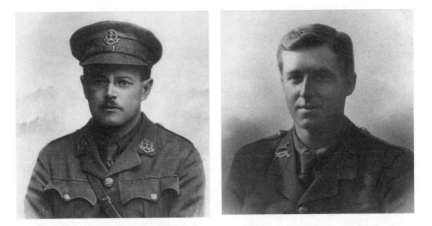

Captain Reginald Underhill (left), Eleventh Middlesex Regiment, and Lieutenant Charles Bertram Underhill, West Yorkshire Regiment, were two of the five Underhill sons who went to war. They were both killed in 1916 at Flanders Fields.

did not permit his grief at the deaths of his sons to intrude on his duties. Circumstances had already conspired to greatly increase his workload because so many doctors and nurses were serving overseas. Now he faced the mysterious, threatening Spanish flu.

On October 1 Underhill received some frightening news out of Seattle and knew the inevitable was only days away. Washington's chief health commissioner, Dr. T.D. Tubble, said the disease was prevalent throughout the state and getting worse as facilities became taxed to the limit. Tubble classified the situation as desperate when he learned that 10 percent of the 1,500 just-arrived sailors at Puget Sound Naval Station were also ill. He told Underhill he was considering a ban on public meetings and all kinds of gatherings to try to contain the disease. Meanwhile, in San Francisco, Dr. Hassler had a number of suspected cases that would grow to 4,000 by mid-October.

One day after his talk with Tubble, Underhill announced that there were no confirmed cases of Spanish flu in Vancouver. He did admit that several people were ill, but said it hadn't yet been confirmed whether it was the ordinary type of winter flu or the new strain that seemed to be so much more dangerous. Other city doctors, however, were quick to diagnose without laboratory confirmation some of their cases as Spanish flu.

In the end, the Spanish Lady crossed into B.C. from Alberta, first appearing in the small mountain community of Corbin. But whether she arrived from the east or the south mattered not. Forty-eight hours later, Vancouver's 110,000 people learned they also were in jeopardy.

All three public health officers took immediate steps to meet the coming crisis. At the provincial level, Dr. Young acted to give municipal health officers around the province more authority. He recommended to the minister of health that municipalities be given the right to make whatever moves they deemed necessary to combat the flu in their own jurisdictions. A simple addition to the regulations gave municipal health officers the authority, at their discretion, to close schools, churches, and places of entertainment—movie halls, theatres, poolrooms, bowling alleys, ballrooms, and the like—for the health of the community.

Young also insisted that the pandemic flu be added to the existing list of contagious diseases. This meant that doctors must report all cases to local health officers, as they did for such things as typhoid or smallpox. He advocated a hefty fine for those who didn't comply. Reporting throughout the pandemic was, however, erratic. Some doctors waited days and then reported a significant number of cases; others reported daily. This caused figures to fluctuate wildly, leading to differing views about whether more people were down with the flu or whether it was on its way out.

Like Dr. Young and Dr. Underhill, Victoria's medical health officer, Dr. Arthur Price, received information from other capital cities across the country. However, the views of the three men on the best measures to take were not always identical. Both Price and Underhill were conscientious medical health officers, doing the best they could with the information at hand, but Price, a little more pompous and rather proud of his position in the capital city and his proximity to the provincial health officer, was often more outspoken and rigid in his approach.

In the much larger city of Vancouver, Underhill's primary concern was to prevent panic. He moved quickly, telling the press that Vancouverites had nothing to fear and would be kept fully informed of the situation. *The Vancouver Daily Sun* on October 5 stated that the disease hit town "quietly, almost stealthily," as Underhill cautiously confirmed the first case. He told reporters plans were in place to meet the attack but had to admit that, like medical authorities around the world, he was uncertain as to what the city was facing. From the outset, his objectives were to calm fears, recommend preventive measures, and find enough beds in isolation hospitals to accommodate the sick and keep them from infecting the rest of the population.

Hospitals prepare for worst

The three public health officers were not alone in their preparations; the administrators of all the major hospitals shared Dr. Underhill's approach. In Vancouver, two important men were preparing to face the epidemic: Dr. Malcolm T. McEachern, the superintendent of Vancouver General Hospital; and his counterpart at St. Paul's, Dr. Francis Xavier McPhillips. McEachern was also superintendent of the Infants' Hospital located in the West End at 1154 Bute Street, where babies less than two years old were treated. For several weeks they had been anticipating the onslaught at the city's two main medical centres, but McEachern reminded hospital doctors and patients that although nobody was sure, flu with a new name didn't necessarily mean a new disease. While admitting that the current outbreak seemed much more virulent than previous ones, he also questioned some of the fatality figures coming in from the east.

Vancouver General Hospital (VGH) was the city's largest hospital, slated to play a major role in fighting the pandemic. The first medical care centre in Vancouver, VGH began in a tent in the Gastown area of the pioneer community. In September 1886, after Vancouver officially became a city, the new Board of Health, in agreement with the Canadian Pacific Railway, established a small building at the corner of Powell Street between Hawkes and Heather. Two years later there was a move to Beatty Street, south of Pender, and a two-storey building that had 35 beds. An operating theatre was built five years later. In 1906 a procession of horse-drawn ambulances containing 47 patients plodded across the plank bridge at False Creek to Heather and Twelfth Avenue, establishing VGH in the same area where the hospital now stands. Today's 1,500 beds make it the second largest in Canada.

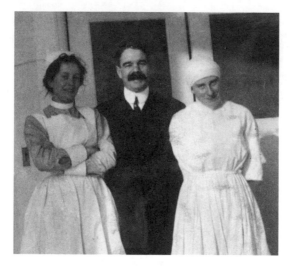

Dr. F.X. McPhillips led the battle against the flu at St. Paul's Hospital in Vancouver. He is pictured here in 1919 with student nurses Dorothy Hutchinson and Kathleen McFarlane.

When the epidemic struck, Dr. McEachern was as ready as he could be. Born in Ontario in 1874, he, like Dr. Young, was a graduate of McGill University, Montreal, in 1910. He was the medical superintendent of Montreal's maternity hospital before moving to the west coast in 1913 and becoming general superintendent of VGH. He undertook a major reorganization of the facility.

St. Paul's Hospital had been operating in Vancouver since 1894, when it was begun by the Sisters of the Charity of Providence, a Catholic order from Montreal. Mother Mary Theresa came to the west coast from Quebec to found it, buying seven lots on the dirt road leading from downtown to English Bay. St Paul's still occupies the same Burrard Street site. By 1906 the hospital had 75 beds, and the following year it introduced its first X-ray machine. The nursing school opened in 1912.

The Sisters of Providence also operated St. Mary's Hospital in New Westminster, which was opened in 1887 by nuns who had come from Washington State. The order went even further, starting the first health-insurance program in B.C.'s history in the late 1890s. Two young nuns on horseback, riding sidesaddle, galloped off through the dense, lonely bush to nearby logging and fishing operations to sign up the workers. For 10 dollars a year, the men bought coverage that would give them admission to hospital; the document a worker received stated that treatment coverage was "in consequence of any disease or injury incapacitating him for labour, except smallpox ... "The Sisters' contract added a stern moralistic caveat, pointing out that coverage did not extend to "cases directly resulting from the use of alcoholic stimulants."

St. Paul's medical superintendent, Dr. McPhillips, was born in Richmond Hill, Ontario, in 1866 and moved with his family to Manitoba after the Riel Rebellion. He graduated from the University of Manitoba in 1889 and came to Vancouver in 1893, working as a doctor for the CPR before going into private practice and then becoming superintendent at St. Paul's.

It was not long before these top Vancouver medical men discovered that it would take their combined efforts and those of every other health-care worker and volunteer in the city to fight off the terrible onslaught now facing them.

Debate on municipal closures begins

There was considerable disagreement in every large North American city on whether or not it was advisable to force closures on downtown businesses. It was much more of a consideration than it would have been if Canada and the U.S. had not been embroiled in fighting World War One. Keeping factories churning out weapons was essential to winning the war. People questioned the effectiveness of a closure that permitted large numbers of people working "in essential services" to carry on as usual, mingling freely and travelling between home and work carrying the infection. If it was only a partial closure, was there any point in enforcing it?

Dr. Price, keeping watch in the capital, knew on October 8 that flu had struck. Even before the first cases were identified he declared, in ringing, patriotic tones, as was his wont: "If Spanish flu should develop we should be bound to use the strongest possible measures to kill the epidemic at once. It would be our duty not only from the national standpoint of public health, but from the duty to Empire." Almost immediately he recommended closing public places in Victoria.

As a small capital city, Victoria's involvement in the war effort was small, and essential services referred only to grocery and drugstores. Victoria City Council debated the issue, and the atmosphere in the chamber was "so hot that no germ could live in it," reported the *Daily Colonist*. Health or business was the crux of the argument, fired by a constant rivalry between Victoria and Vancouver. The capital's businessmen knew that Fred Underhill had made no recommendations for closure in Vancouver, and they were leery of anything that might give the mainland city such an economic advantage. Nonetheless, Price's forceful viewpoint carried the day, no doubt helped by the more astute members of council who, while having their doubts, did not want to put themselves in the position of being blamed for illness and death.

The *Colonist* reported on the first night of the closures that "the streets were deserted and the few people who populated them drifted about aimlessly and peevishly." At the same time, drugstores were running out of the cinnamon bark they flogged for fending off the flu.

Libraries soon recorded a record number of book loans. Surprisingly, many schoolchildren were said to be worried about an unexpected holiday because they were losing time before year-end exams, which were only short weeks away. Some young men with immediate plans for marriage pleaded for churches to be kept open, but Price refused. He was equally adamant with prominent visitors, refusing to allow a meeting between four federal ministers and local politicians that was scheduled at the Canadian Club. This angered Victoria businessmen, who knew that their Vancouver rivals, in a larger and more industrialized city, would capitalize on the exclusive chance to lobby the national ministers.

In Vancouver, Dr. Underhill had confirmed five flu cases by October 8, but expected all of the victims to recover. He stressed that it had been difficult to confirm whether the patients were suffering from ordinary flu or the Spanish variety and added that severe cases would be taken immediately to an isolation hospital for full care. In keeping with his preventative approach to fighting the flu, he had recommended that a major information campaign be undertaken to put people on their guard. Nothing had come of his suggestion, but after a meeting with Vancouver Mayor Harry Gale, Underhill issued a list of do's and don'ts for the public, which was printed in the newspapers. The mayor said the city had a "trap ready to be sprung at a minute's notice if the attack became serious," although exactly what he meant wasn't clear. He likely was referring to Underhill's preparations or perhaps to the possibility of closing down the city's non-essential services.

The mayor was a transplanted Montrealer who came to Vancouver in 1910 and went into business as a marble contractor. An ambitious entrepreneur, he was barely 40 when he ran for an aldermanic seat and won, surprising some because of his fairly recent arrival on the coast. He was a smooth talker and a good political campaigner and by early 1918 had attained the mayor's post.

Up to this point, Underhill had experienced difficulty trying to get the city fathers to prepare for the Spanish Lady's arrival. Gale was now anxious to be seen doing the right thing and suggested closing down the schools, as Price had done in Victoria. Underhill spoke strongly against this, but did agree diplomatically with Gale's proposal to ask places of entertainment to voluntarily keep children out.

It was also agreed that Underhill would make daily reports to the press. In an era when the bureaucracy was even keener on holding information as close as possible to its chest than it is today, this was a slightly radical move. But despite being 60, the medical chief wasn't dyed-in-the-wool. He knew the value of public relations and how to get his message across, and he was respected and liked by people in the newspaper business.

Underhill was opposed to closing schools unless the situation deteriorated badly because he felt that teachers and school administrators could keep a better eye on children if they were in school rather than free to wander the streets and gather on street corners. He knew well that hard-pressed mothers were managing on their own while their husbands were away at the front, single-handedly operating many households. Many of these women worked in factories and tried to look after their families at night. They were frequently short of money; large families were common in this era. Underhill knew it would be an additional hardship to these mothers if he closed the schools.

81

When there was near panic after reports came in of a large number of children down with flu—Laura Secord School at 2500 Lakewood was hard hit—Underhill hurried to make a public statement. He assured residents that only 300 of 16,000 students in all city schools were off with colds and assorted minor complaints, and suggested that some parents were keeping their children home needlessly. His concerns, he said, were focused on men and women between 20 and 45 years of age, the age group already identified in other parts of Canada and in many other countries as most susceptible to the Spanish flu.

Dr. Robert Wightman, the medical officer for schools, supported Underhill and said there was still no need to close. In fact, he said, a study comparing September 1917 and September 1918 showed that absenteeism was lower in the year of the epidemic. This, of course, was almost a moot point, as the Spanish flu did not arrive until October.

Meanwhile, on the commercial side, Vancouver businessmen watched developments in Victoria with some apprehension, and owners of non-essential services like theatres and bowling alleys worried about impending closures. Their city was a hive of activity as war work continued, and money made by the men and women employed there kept cash registers clanging. They had heard the anguished cries of their Victoria counterparts, even though newspapers there reported that "peace and solitude reigned" in the provincial capital.

Fred Underhill, always the diplomat, knew any precipitous moves on his part would meet with criticism and hostility, possibly increasing the general level of conflict, apprehension, and fear. His political colleagues, Mayor Gale and the city fathers, were concerned about the need to juggle their responsibilities for public health with the need to keep the city operating. Moreover, Underhill had studied the results of general closures in the U.S. and knew that such action had mixed results. He asked, "Should we seek permission from Victoria to save the people from themselves or leave them to exercise their own free will and common sense to go or stay away as they see fit?" He did strongly advise staying away from crowds when possible, adding somewhat testily that he couldn't understand why women "pottered" around stores when they didn't have to. He sniffed and noted they probably had wet feet, too.

The newspapers strongly backed Underhill in his campaign for prevention rather than closure. Several local doctors expressed pro-closure views when Winnipeg reported that it was shutting down, but they were taken to task by city physician H.B. Gourlay, who said private medical men should not be offering opinions because "there are many others better placed and informed to know what is developing."

On October 9, Underhill faced a quandary. Should he shut everything down as Victoria had done? Only one thing was now abundantly clear: The death toll was mounting everywhere, including in Victoria. Young was receiving reports from all over the province showing that the number of cases and deaths was climbing, both on the coast and in the interior.

Advice and treatment

Vancouver's defence was already in place. Underhill had long ago ensured clean water and pasteurized milk for residents. His reporting regulations and system of quarantine signs were accepted as standard procedure, and they became assets in controlling the disease. During October and November 1918, the quarantine signs proliferated everywhere in the city. In most cases, the large yellow posters simply kept visitors away, but they were also the source of some fear and concern. It was not a heartening sight when nearly every house on the block boasted a contagious-disease sign.

Underhill also offered advice to individuals, starting with a stern warning to the people of Vancouver: "Don't play the fool." He advised everyone to go to bed as soon as they experienced any symptoms, be it a temperature, cough, aches, or chills. He stressed the need for ventilation in the home and said sick patients should be fed wholesome food, if they felt up to eating.

When two sick people were in the same room, Underhill suggested a sheet be hung between the beds to minimize the direct effect of coughing and sneezing. He also advised caregivers to place gauze over their noses and mouths when they were in the same room with their patients. A man of his era, sedate, dignified, and conservative, Dr. Underhill also suggested that young women not bow to some of the new fashion trends—the latest dictates of style, he said, which had produced "high skirts and low waists," were invitations to colds and flu.

In advocating prevention as the best defence, he issued a list of do's and don'ts for children. He wrote in simple language that they could readily understand.

- Use hankies.
- Don't borrow a hankie and don't lend yours to anyone else.
- Don't spit.
- Don't take a lick of anybody else's sucker.
- Don't take a bite of a friend's apple.
- Don't bite the end of your pencil.
- Don't lick your marbles.
- Keep your feet dry and out of dirty water.
- Keep windows open.
- Swat flies, because they carry disease.
- Save your pennies and keep away from crowded picture halls.
- Keep desks tidy.
- Don't leave hankies around, keep them in your pocket.

As a father of 13, he knew well youngsters and their reactions. Of his recommendations, he said, "Take them to heart. Play the game, and help us to drive Spanish flu from Vancouver."

Underhill prepared an equivalent list of precautions for adults; some were more easily said than done. They included:

- Avoid such public places as movie halls and streetcars.
- Avoid people suffering colds, coughs, and sore throats.
- Sleep and work in clean fresh air.
- Be in a premises not below 68 degrees and not above 72 degrees.
- Keep hands clean and well away from the mouth.
- Don't spit.
- Avoid visiting anyone who is sick.
- Eat plain, nourishing food.
- Keep off alcohol.

- Use hankies, and boil soiled ones.
- Keep feet warm.
- Don't worry.

These suggestions were carried in all the newspapers. The mayor and council also issued an authorized list of recommendations developed by Dr. Underhill. These were: Try to keep away from other people; don't kiss anybody; use individual dishes and utensils; if symptoms occur, go to bed immediately and stay in bed for three days after symptoms disappear. Bank tellers were warned to be sure that the water they used to wet their thumbs while counting money contained antiseptic.

To the chagrin of some druggists, Underhill also stated in one newspaper report: "There is no specific [medicine] for the disease, and symptoms should be met as they arise." He added that the great danger was pneumonia, which could develop as symptoms seemed to improve, hence the need for full convalescence. The after-effects, he said, could be much worse than the flu itself.

From the point of view of modern physicians, Underhill's advice was generally sound and sometimes ahead of his time. It was even more remarkable considering the wide divergence of medical opinion that soon developed over almost every aspect of recommended treatment for flu patients. The medical officer in Saanich, Victoria's neighbour, took a simple view, recommending that "everybody should get out as much as possible into God's fresh air," while others recommended the opposite: "Stay home, keep warm, and stay out of drafts."

In England, Dr. C. Stennett of Trafford Hall Hospital, Manchester, advocated a treatment that was readily acceptable to his patients even if it cured nothing. He gave them 16 grams of salicylate of soda with two spoonfuls of the very best Scotch whiskey in very hot water every three to four hours. He claimed that the results "were phenomenal and I have never adopted any other line of treatment." If Stennett's patients weren't cured, at least they were happy.

In Mount Pleasant, a residential suburb of Vancouver, William N. De Page had a solution of his own that he said had worked in his considerable experience in dealing with grippe. It called for putting in each shoe enough sulphur to cover a dime. Another doctor advocated eating three cakes of yeast a day, while a woman contended that the answer was to gargle with three drops of crude carbolic.

Doctors were equally divided on the efficacy of a new and scarce vaccine. The few doses available had been given to doctors and nurses, largely with the belief that they might do some good and wouldn't do any harm. Many members of the public were clamouring to know more and asking to get shots as soon as new supplies arrived from eastern Canada. Later evidence indicated that the shots were of little help.

Those trying to treat the flu at home resorted to patent medicines, few of which were of any use. Canadian medicine cabinets of the time contained little more than sugar syrup for coughs and colds, Epsom salts, the usual cod-liver oil tonic, and, without doubt, the dreaded bottle of castor oil. Assuming it was safer to try an old and trusted remedy than ignore the situation, some people wore bags of strong-smelling camphor around their necks. They burned foul-smelling bouquets in the hope that the fumes would ward off the disease, sniffed saltwater to clear their sinuses, or drank a mixture of milk, ginger, sugar, and soda to ease a sore throat. One rather noxious preventive was tea laced with mustard, a concoction that would make anyone gag. Steaming-hot poultices of many kinds were slapped on chests.

Potions and elixirs pushed by drugstores and travelling apothecaries were seldom useful as preventives or cures for anything, but were often purchased by a population that felt it was better to be safe than sorry. Many of the outrageous products of the era's snake-oil salesmen benefited only the profiteers who flogged them.

Some companies developed public measures of their own to help their customers combat the flu. B.C. Electric Railway in Vancouver told streetcar conductors to tell passengers to keep car windows open, regardless of the drafts that howled in. The company said fresh air was essential to combat the spread of the flu. To ease the fears of passengers and to encourage more people to use the cars, already frequently packed at morning and evening rush hours, BCER announced that it would fumigate the cars every day instead of about once every two weeks as was customary. The company also hoped that the powerful smell of the mixture of formaldehyde and permanganate of potash would provide reassurance rather than revulsion. During the epidemic, disinfectants that smelled strongly were preferred in order to remind people of the need for preventive measures.

One bicycle company's advertisement urged people to take up cycling as a fresh-air alternative to the crowded public-transit system and as an opportunity to build themselves up through exercise. Advice in advertisements that companies placed was often mixed with statements of confidence in the public's ability to weather the storm—along with a fair amount of commercial self-interest.

During the early days of the outbreak, a couple of small poems making the rounds took a light-hearted approach to the whole situation. They read:

> A flea and a fly had the flu,
> They neither were sure what to do,
> "Let's fly," said the flea,
> "Let us flee," said the fly,
> So they went away through a flaw in the flue.

> There was a little bird,
> Its name was Enza,
> I opened the window,
> And in flew Enza.

The Vancouver Daily Sun told its readers that the epidemic hadn't fared too well when it hit Vancouver, as though it was some kind of contest. It said there had been a barrage of disinfectants, regulations, and advice, along with "intelligent" conferences about ways to combat the flu, and contended that residents were well informed. The message may have come from Dr. Underhill, still anxious to calm unnecessary fears. The paper quoted him as stating that carelessness in personal and public hygiene was the greatest danger, and that every case of flu should be treated as serious and every known precaution taken.

Asked about the upcoming heavy rains typical of a Vancouver fall, Underhill said downpours represented "one of the finest cleaning agents." *The Sun* said the health officer was cool-headed and refused to be stampeded "by the first germ that tries to rush his sanitary defences." The paper also stated that there had been unnecessary efforts to frighten the populace and force closure of public institutions. In this, it may also have had an eye on its own business, its readership and advertisers.

In Victoria, when the sun shone, Dr. Price expressed the view that it might help to discourage the disease from spreading further. One *Colonist* reporter got carried away and wrote, "Several hours of bright sunshine landed a staggering blow on the Spanish flu epidemic in Victoria yesterday. A few more hours of it today and tomorrow will probably result in a knock out."

Mayor Gale hurried to say that most of the Vancouver cases involved people from outside coming into the city, although what point he was trying to make was rather obscure; possibly it was just the jitters of a new mayor with a critical crisis on his hands.

The Vancouver Relief Department's George P. Ireland was also in the sanguine camp. "No great danger exists if proper precautions are taken," he told reporters, confidently adding, "I think we will pull through this epidemic without much loss of life and crippling activity, serious as the situation undoubtedly is." Ireland also said restaurants and theatres were being fumigated daily, although local manufacturers were having trouble keeping up with the demand for strong-smelling creosote or Lysol.

As items used for treatment ran short, commercial interest became stronger. Lemons in particular were thought to be good for warding off the flu, and prices shot up as supplies became scarce. There were many who saw an opportunity to make money from the epidemic and started to push their wares.

Among the first was the Vancouver Drug Company. It advertised: "Safeguard Yourself against Spanish flu. Take Reid's Grip-Fix pills, 35-cents-a-box." There were buyers for these, as well as for all the other so-called remedies and potions offered to the public. An unctuous advertisement by Burns Drug Company warned readers about "unscrupulous people trying to benefit from misfortune." It was doing exactly the same thing, however, touting its own wares with false claims that they either staved off or prevented flu. Burns stated that the Regal-brand prescriptions it carried had done well in England and the U.S. Its large ad in local papers read: "Burns Compound Cinnamon

Tablets, not the same as the ordinary ones, special: Regal Essence of Cinnamon—for relief of and cure of Spanish Flu, discovered in the laboratory of M. Pasteur of Paris that the microbe of the disease of influenza was rendered inert by this essence: Cinnamon Compound Tablet, for the prevention of Spanish Flu."

Also touted in one of the newspapers was Kennedy's Tonic Port, said to be "the great South American remedy whose chief ingredient was the Conchona Tree bark, written about first by Sebastien Babos (1663) and endorsed by eminent physicians and sold by druggists."

Underhill and his colleagues knew the claims were nonsense, but didn't denounce these self-proclaimed panaceas. The doctors probably took the view that if these concoctions made people think they were being helped, they weren't doing any harm.

A RELENTLESS FOE DIGS IN

While public views on the pandemic swung between dire pessimism and optimistic hope, the Spanish flu took hold everywhere, and apprehension turned into tragedy.

During the first week of the flu in Vancouver, 72 cases were reported to Dr. Underhill and the first two deaths were recorded—low numbers compared to many other cities. It was, however, only the beginning, and by the 10-day mark, hospital staffs were hard pressed to cope with the influx of patients. Physicians and nurses were working 16-hour shifts and a bed shortage loomed. By day 11 there were 100 more cases than there were the day before, and another two deaths. Vancouver had 200 reported cases by October 14, and it was feared that many other people were sick but hadn't seen a doctor. Seven people were dead.

Despite the extra closures and restrictions, in Victoria there were almost 200 reported cases, with about 40 in hospital. Dr. Price continued to deny permits for all public gatherings, even church weddings planned months earlier. He also cautioned girls in Victoria against kissing sailors.

Newspaper accounts in October suggest that in Victoria in particular there remained some reluctance on the part of editors to publish the actual number of the sick and the dead. By October 15, however, Victorians knew there had been 230 reported cases, and two days later the figure soared to 525. Official hopes dimmed as the disease spread like wildfire through the capital city.

Point Grey municipality on the mainland reported only six cases during the first two weeks of October. It was an area of single-family homes, without the abundance of boarding houses that seemed to be the flu's prime breeding ground in Vancouver. A similar situation existed in the municipality of South Vancouver, where the number of initial cases was smaller. Soon, however, both municipalities began to count more cases. North Vancouver decided to close its schools, but the shipyards were operating at full capacity, and any victims of the flu were being sent to Vancouver hospitals.

In order to accommodate hospital crowding, which occurred within a day or two of the outbreak, Vancouver city officials and leading medical men conferred and decided to take over the auditorium and adjacent classrooms at the University of British Columbia. The original UBC buildings, known as the King Edward campus, were close to VGH and were quickly converted into an isolation unit for the sole purpose of treating flu cases during the crisis.

In Victoria, two additional emergency hospitals were set up. The first was the old Victoria Hotel, which was taken over and equipped with extra beds and sheets; the second was an old fire hall, which was quickly pressed into service when the hotel almost instantly became overcrowded.

The fact that Vancouver remained wide open soon brought protests from closed communities nearby, and the provincial government began to feel the increased pressure. S.D. MacLean, the minister responsible for health, indicated he might have to take action to force closure on Vancouver. Underhill continued to voice his opposition, and his arguments for staying open, together with his long service to and stature in the community, carried considerable weight, but many elected city officials were becoming nervous because voters worried about catching the flu were asking about the lack of closure.

War effort takes priority

With no sign that Dr. Price's strategy was any more effective than Dr. Underhill's, Mayor Gale announced that a planned late-October Thanksgiving service in downtown Vancouver would go ahead. He said the event at Georgia and Gilford streets would celebrate the recent military victories in the war, where the end was now in sight. It would also be an opportunity to pray for the success of the upcoming national Victory Loan campaign. The mayor said organizers were taking every precaution and would ensure "the Spanish flu will not be spread, every door and window will be open and disinfectant spread." Throughout the pandemic, Victory Loan campaigns and the obvious patriotism of the population were much in evidence, the fundraisers and military reports nearly always taking precedence over the latest news about the flu.

Although in retrospect it seems a ludicrous decision, the mayor knew his audience and was preparing for re-election. He also approved a mass rally in support of the National Victory Loan Drive, and the committee in charge immediately began planning a huge downtown parade that would encourage crowds to gather along the main streets. Their first project was preparing 354 flags that would decorate lamp standards.

On October 28, only two weeks after the mayor had given his approval, the loan drive drew a large crowd. Civic authorities had urged the public not to congregate, yet they also called on everyone to come downtown for the opening ceremonies. Factory and ship whistles blew and church bells rang as Mayor Gale signed the city's $1-million cheque, taken from reserve funds to buy bonds. The national goal was $500 million and Vancouver's target was $15 million.

The country needed the money badly to pay the costs of fighting the war, to help resettle hundreds of thousands of veterans, and to finance the replacement of utilities ignored for four long years. Campaign chairman W.H. Malkin told the crowd: "Let us tell the Kaiser and the Germans that Canada can fight and means to put an end to the Kaiser forever." Spectators whistled appreciatively as Empress Theatre vaudeville artist Lottie Fletcher, dressed appropriately in khaki, scaled a fire department hook-and-ladder unit to hang a campaign banner across the front of the city hall. And nobody worried much about catching the flu.

About the same time, another event drew a large number of cheering well-wishers to the downtown area. These participants, too, ignored warnings about avoiding crowds and filled the CPR station

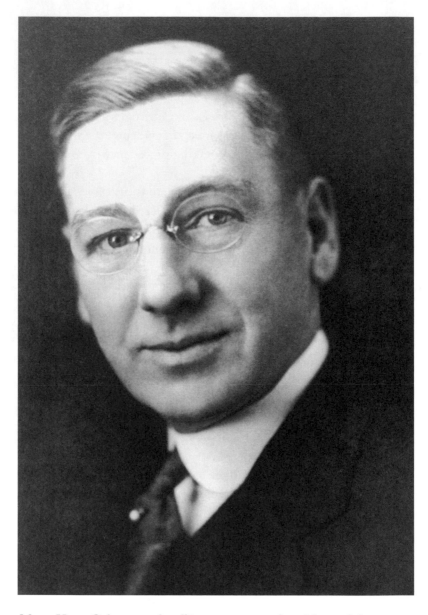

Mayor Harry Gale, a smooth-talking entrepreneur from Montreal, became Vancouver's mayor in 1918, working with Dr. Underhill and city council to fight the frightening epidemic that nearly brought the city to a standstill.

to welcome home more than 200 veterans arriving from France. The Vancouver *Daily Province* reported that many vets were on crutches or limping, and showing the pallor picked up in hospital wards or in German prisoner-of-war camps. "Wounded, ill, happy to be home, one left two brothers buried in France," the paper stated. Sadly, in the next few weeks more of them would die from the Spanish flu. They were among the young men who suffered most severely, susceptible because of their poor physical condition.

Visiting federal finance minister Sir Thomas White welcomed the men. He said that although Canada had suffered the heavy cost of war, signs of increasing national unity were apparent. He admitted that part of the price paid was the death of nine soldiers at military hospitals in Coquitlam and in Fairmont, in the B.C. interior, where there were now some 300 patients.

Never wavering under fire, the doughty Dr. Underhill was now working extremely long hours, spending hectic days and nights with little time for sleep. He always appeared confident, cheerful, and well turned-out, but as the flu ravaged the city, new problems developed.

Underhill said that loggers and miners arriving for temporary stays in the city were now creating Vancouver's biggest problem. Some of them were ailing when they arrived, others were not. He said they chose lodgings in the oldest part of town, going to "low-down rooming houses in certain areas where there is but one sitting room and where they sit around the stove smoking and spitting freely." The doctor maintained that under these conditions it was almost impossible for any of them to escape the clutches of the Spanish Lady.

During one of his daily briefings to the press, he declared that in the poorer parts of town, rooming houses were over-crowded, poorly maintained, cold, drafty, and dirty. He wanted to remove the sick from these premises and transfer them to hospitals, where they could be assured of warmth and proper food, increasing their chances of survival.

He explained that conventional medicines that could ease a patient's discomfort were available in hospitals. Quinine was of some use, he said, and nurses could try to bring down temperatures by applying cold compresses, or, by applying heat, relieve some of the terrible aches and soreness that accompanied the Spanish flu. Hot poultices were slapped on chests to relieve congestion, and so many had been applied that an urgent appeal went out for donations of linen and other materials needed to make them.

Underhill also issued a notice telling operators of hotels, lodgings, and rooming houses that they were required by law to ensure medical attention for any sick person on their premises. They were also required to report any case of the flu to the city health department; he reminded Vancouverites that these rules applied to anyone who had sickness in their home.

Call for volunteers goes out

As the caseload increased, nurses found their ranks depleted as they, too, contracted the Spanish flu in large numbers, despite their wearing gowns and masks that covered them from head to toe. One doctor said it was a rather eerie sight in dimly lit wards at night to see these white apparitions floating through a sea of tightly packed, white-quilted beds.

It was not long before the first of many calls went out for volunteers to help in hospitals. In this instance, as well as in many other later calls for help, there was a mixed response. Some women came forward readily to do what they could; others hesitated for fear of contracting the flu themselves; still others were so afraid, they all but shut themselves in their homes, seeing no one.

In addition to hospital duties, volunteers were often assigned to homes in which all of the adults were prostrate. It was not an easy job, particularly for some of the younger women, who quickly lost their eagerness to help when they found themselves in ramshackle, dirty houses where they were expected to wash and diaper ragged, runny-nosed children on top of cleaning up after adult patients who could do nothing for themselves.

Vancouver relief department's George Ireland also put out calls for husky teenagers to come to the hospitals to help with some of the heavy lifting and carrying. Ireland made the request on behalf of Dr. McEachern, who had now closed the VGH to all visitors because of the shortage of trained personnel and in hopes that it would slow the spread of the virulent pandemic. Hospitals were having considerable difficulty coping with the increasing number of patients.

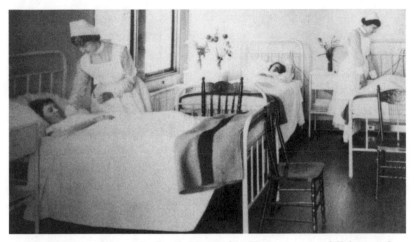

A ward for sick nurses at St. Paul's Hospital in Vancouver was full during the epidemic

McEachern made a special appeal to the city's wealthy citizens, saying that the wartime military demand had badly cut the number of available nurses. He asked the well-to-do ladies to release anyone they had hired for their personal needs, as these women were more urgently needed in hospitals. The doctor said that despite some problems, the health services were well organized to meet this challenge, and that "I feel with the precautions that have been taken, the flu will be kept under control."

Mayor Gale paid tribute to those who did come forward to help but had harsh words for those who could render help but didn't. He said Vancouver expected more of its people in a time of crisis. His words shamed some into volunteering.

Dr. Price announced a great shortage of nurses in Victoria and pleaded for volunteers. In his own patriotic style, he suggested that the situation gave people a chance "to render service not only to their city but to the country. Here is a chance to fight a formidable foe right in your own home." All that was needed, he said, "was a good head and a pair of hands." He was a man with his own ideas about cause and treatment and took credit for the city's actions in adopting his closing policy, claiming that it held back the flu. Price also stated that an overnight "rain had chased a good many flu germs into the gutter and stopped the chance of dying in Victoria."

Price's closure policy hadn't shut down all business in Victoria. Life-insurance companies in particular were doing a bustling trade, and while it would be difficult to categorize life insurance as an essential service, the need for insurance was obvious and offices were open and flourishing. One spokesman said he was "issuing dozens of policies and for every $24 invested, a victim's beneficiary would be paid $1,000." But if sales were growing, payouts were also mounting. Prudential Life Assurance superintendent Charles Preston said that in Vancouver his company had received at least 50 claims in the past two weeks for flu deaths. A Merchants Casualty Company spokesman reported that that company had received 110 claims.

The crisis worsens

Unfortunately, there was little co-operation among communities in the Lower Mainland and throughout the province in fighting the disease; they had always functioned separately. This same situation prevailed nationally. Some public health officials and politicians co-operated, as was the case in Vancouver and Victoria, but the co-operation was often hard fought for and short-lived. It would have helped if surrounding municipalities had been brought into the picture, but it had never been done before and would have been difficult to organize in the middle of a crisis situation. Most city and municipal politicians had their own ideas of the best procedures, which they touted independently to their own constituents.

During one debate in the House of Commons it was stressed that there was no organization in the country to oversee the flu crisis. Members were told that the situation was being left to local individuals, many of them ill informed and all of them lacking in co-ordinated effort. This was one of the earliest public intimations in Parliament that the country was badly in need of a national body to oversee public health in Canada.

News from Washington, D.C., said U.S. health authorities were trying to find a vaccine that would be effective, but noted that "the service has as yet been unable to recommend any that it deduced will be successful." This supported the view held by many B.C. doctors: The vaccine they had administered to medical staff was a morale booster but not much more.

As the crisis worsened and the number of cases began to increase dramatically, Mayor Gale called a special meeting of city council that included leading medical authorities and allied groups. Underhill again found himself defending his position on closure. He received the full support of the group when he pointed out that some similar-sized communities that had shut down were reporting more cases and deaths than was Vancouver.

Mayor Gale, his eye still on the next election, said he didn't think the public supported Underhill's position, but he was alone in this view. Underhill, an older and more respected long-term resident, had the backing of most aldermen, as well as the Vancouver Medical Association, the school board, and the board of the Vancouver General Hospital. Stressing that it was acting strictly on Underhill's advice, council passed a carefully worded resolution:

> The action of the medical officer in his stand
> against closing down schools, places of public
> entertainment, etc., at present, has been approved
> as being a step, in his opinion, which would
> by no means eradicate the evil, but might have
> the adverse effect, especially among the school
> children, who would no doubt more or less run
> at large on city streets with every possibility of
> accentuating the possibility.

It certainly was not a very clear and concise resolution, and it contained enough weasel words to place the blame squarely on Underhill should the situation worsen. These were elected officials with their own reputations at stake. Nobody knew better than the steadfast Underhill what he could expect from them.

On October 16, less than two weeks into the pandemic, the caseload in Vancouver had grown to 400, with 13 people dead and several patients who had developed pneumonia close to death. Pressure mounted steadily for closures. Leaders of several surrounding locations complained that while some precautions had been taken, Vancouver was operating as usual and outsiders coming into town had an increased chance of contracting the disease. It was a specious argument, but with the death toll mounting, fear needed little rationale. So many were now ill that closures in unusual areas were becoming common. There was even a temporary courtroom closure when jurors fell ill. And worse was yet to come.

Influx from coast

While doctors organized the best treatment they could devise, Mayor Gale and Vancouver City Council tried to deal with a major new problem: A dramatic increase in the number of small boats arriving in the city from upcoast communities and carrying flu victims, some very ill, some already dead. There were many sad, sombre scenes along the waterfront as blanket-covered corpses were carried ashore. Some victims had travelled for days and suffered terribly in the hope of finding the medical help they needed. These people, and those from some of the larger boats like the *Venture,* which had arrived with nine patients, added to the pressure on VGH and St. Paul's. The mayor said the province should attempt to establish another temporary upcoast hospital where victims of the flu could be taken instead of suffering through the long voyage to Vancouver. However, there were no buildings available and no trained staff to minister to the sick. Nothing could be done.

The provincial government owed some concern to these mid-coast settlers: In conjunction with the Union Steamship Company, it had for over a year been promoting land sales and new settlement. The province had offered 160-acre parcels of land free if they were occupied for six months of the year and cleared and planted. Title to the land would be granted after five years if these conditions were met, and a large number of young people with families had taken up the offer. Many of these isolated settlers now needed medical help. It was left to Columbia Coast Mission hospitals and boats to cope with the crisis. Although for many years the tiny coastal settlements between Prince Rupert and Vancouver—logging and construction camps, as well as small farming communities—had not had any medical facilities, they did receive regular visits from two dedicated Anglican ministers. Since 1910, the church's Columbia Coast Mission had ministered to the medical and spiritual needs of B.C.'s coastal pioneers. Reverend John Antle founded the service and was soon joined by Reverend Alan Greene. They sailed on two ships, making regular runs to these isolated settlements, and in time they established three small hospitals.

Their first ship, *John Antle*, had originally sported a naked painted lady; she was removed from the bow before the vessel set sail on her new mission. The second, the 106-ton *Columbia*, plied the coastal waters for almost 50 years. The *John Antle* was retired in the 1930s. There were also Columbia Coast Mission hospitals: St. Mary's at Pender Harbour; St. Michael's at Rock Bay; and St. George's Hospital at Alert Bay. The mission itself was headquartered at Valdes, now Quadra Island.

Reverend Greene was known in every small community on the coast. He conducted church services, filled shopping orders, and entertained whenever he was asked to on a folding pump organ that he played by ear and took ashore for services. He sang lustily and often.

During the pandemic, Reverend Antle praised the hospital doctors and nurses who struggled to deal with an ever-increasing number of cases. He said St. Michael's "had a full share of it and for

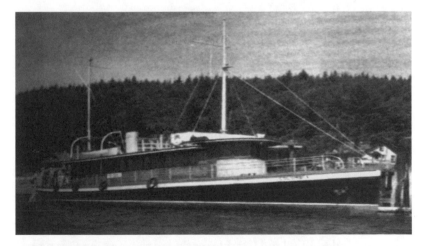

During the Spanish flu epidemic, the Columbia Coast Mission hospital ship Columbia *brought assistance to small, isolated coastal communities that had no medical facilities.*

a while was in great straits. One of the nurses, Alisa Fry, died and the hospital matron took to her bed, leaving Dr. Sutherland alone at the over-full hospital." Antle knew the small communities would need extra help: "the epidemic will visit all the small settlements during the winter, and as most of them are far from medical aid, the hospital boat *Columbia* is being fitted out with everything necessary to help and will sail again for the coast in a few days."

Some central-coast victims feared the *Columbia* would not arrive in time and made their own way to Vancouver, only to die en route. This added measurably to the almost-daily funeral processions winding their way through downtown streets. Businessmen hurrying to their next appointment often stopped two or three times within a few blocks to doff their hats, as was the custom of the day, in tribute to a passing cortege. The city had lived with death all through the war years, but the black horses and processions of mourners constantly reminded those who saw them that they might be the next victims of this unstoppable illness. There was soon a severe shortage of gravediggers, and even wages of $4 per day had not enticed enough volunteers to take on this job.

Closure debate continues

Another special meeting of city council was called. Various large city organizations were invited, including the Board of Trade, the Manufacturers' Association, the Rotary Club, and labour and women's organizations. Underhill reviewed the situation, explaining that the city's medical resources were stretched to the limit trying to cope with an influx of patients from outside. He said 15 new patients had been taken off a steamer from Prince Rupert and more were arriving hourly from near and far. Alderman Joseph Hoskins said council should decide what to do without getting opinions from groups with special interests, while Alderman Frank Woodside cautioned against doing anything "panicky."

Mayor Gale repeated that the responsibility for the city's actions rested on Underhill's shoulders. He reminded the meeting that he and council had acted strictly on medical advice. He said it laughingly, but it was more the smile of the crocodile. Knowing he could be left taking the blame, Dr. Underhill said he was well aware of all the ramifications, adding, "I believe we have got ahead of it at the present time judging by the way the reporting of cases stands tonight." Mayor Gale decided to support his health officer one more time. He pointed out that Winnipeg had ordered widespread closures but still had more cases than Vancouver, while New York City had close to 3,000 dead as flu continued there unabated, despite its shutdowns.

Alderman Frederick P. Rogers threw what *The Daily Province* described as a "bombshell" during the two-hour meeting when he said that 1,887 schoolchildren were absent that day. The actual flu figure wasn't clear, but it was thought to be low because worried parents were acting on their own to keep children at home.

J.H. McVety, representing the Trades and Labour Council, said no thought should be given to closing buildings or plants that had good ventilation. A manufacturers' spokesman, knowing Underhill's views, recommended giving the health officer full discretionary powers.

An unexpected opposing view came from a Vancouver Medical Association spokesman, who now said that all schools should be closed immediately. He even questioned the wisdom of bringing together the 100 people to whom he was speaking. A ministerial association representative favoured closing all public places.

VGH's Dr. McEachern came out against closure because "human psychology gives idle people time to believe they are sick when they are not." Another spokesman opposed anything that could throw Vancouver into a panic, a simmering possibility when more and more people were getting sick and dying, and yellow quarantine signs were appearing in ever-increasing numbers. After much inconclusive debate, the groups decided unanimously that the future course of action should be the joint responsibility of city council, the health board, and the school board. For the moment Vancouver remained open.

With municipalities all around him closing, Underhill continued to stick to his position. His main opposition was to school closures; he still firmly believed that children were better off in school than roaming the streets or confined to homes with sick parents. His view did worry Victoria officials, and provincial secretary S.D. MacLean, who was responsible for health, said he was sending Dr. Young to check out the situation.

Mayor Gale took time out to present bronze badges to 88 "soldiers of the soil," students of King Edward High School who had participated in a food-growing program. The epidemic was having a direct effect on agricultural production, which was already suffering from a lack of manpower because of the war. In one case, Phyllis Hill-Tout, 19, formerly of Vancouver, had struggled with her three younger brothers to maintain the family farm at Abbotsford. When she caught the flu, she died.

Suddenly it seemed that the situation was much worse everywhere. More than 400 Victorians were reported ailing, and in Vancouver the number of cases jumped sharply to 758. Forty victims arrived from logging camps. The ranks of police and fire departments were depleted as members fell ill and took to their beds. Cargo ships in Vancouver were being tied up at berths and left there because there were not enough longshoremen on their feet to load and unload them. City fathers worried about their ability to cope with any fresh disaster.

The outbreak was decimating Vancouver's young male population, including four men who had left only weeks before with the ambition of becoming fliers. Percy Archambeault had been in the service for only a month when flu claimed him at a base in Toronto. Gerald Miles Harvey, 18, an only son said to have a great future ahead of him, had been gone for only three weeks when he wrote home to say that he had the flu, but was recovering. He died, as did Germain Pallen, who had gone east four months earlier, and 26-year-old law student Greenan A. Davidson, son of pioneer merchant C.N. Davidson.

The roll call went on. Alan Maitland Harper, aged 20, was the only son of Dr. Edward E. Harper, a well-known Vancouver composer, pianist, and organist. He had taken a job with the United Grain Growers in Calgary and then become ill, dying on Christmas Day, 1918.

Mrs. R.A. Mather of Vancouver died of flu while visiting Niagara Falls, leaving behind a husband and two small children. North Vancouver recorded the death of the six-year-old son of Mr. and Mrs. John Symonds. The Spanish Lady took them all.

In New Westminster, Dr. S.C. McEwan said he had 50 flu cases and two deaths and announced that he was closing places of entertainment. Restaurants would stay open, he said, but patrons were advised to eat quickly and leave promptly. Dishes and utensils were to be well washed, and all hotels and rooming houses would be inspected. The doctor said that Red Cross rooms would remain open "where the work is of such patriotic nature that it must go on."

Vancouver's problems coping with the influx of upcoast patients were compounded when 100 sick miners arrived by boat from Britannia. As pleas for help poured in from the outlying areas, there was little to offer either in the way of trained medical personnel or medicine. A doctor and two nurses, however, volunteered for the long trip to the Queen Charlottes, and three medical orderlies were sent to Thurston Island in answer to a desperate call for help for 150 victims there. There are no tallies of how many died unattended or with help from people who had care and concern but no medical experience.

In Vancouver, a Dr. Takawara and two others were praised for their independence and performance in treating members of the local Japanese community. They opened a clinic in a mission hall on Powell Street as an emergency hospital staffed by Japanese nurses.

There were so many bizarre stories during the crisis that few could cause surprise, although *The Daily Province* carried one that stretched credibility. The report contended that well-known Lillooet mining man Tom Lewis had been struck down while alone in a cabin 6,000 feet up a local mountain. After five days without a fire or much food, he supposedly struggled down the mountain and back to civilization. When Lewis arrived at Lillooet, his flu had disappeared. Another tall story, unsupported by any B.C. doctor, claimed that smoking could help beat the flu. It was touted that tobacco smoke would kill germs in the lungs. There was little knowledge then about the connection between smoking and lung cancer, and no doubt the theory caused some people to puff harder, more often.

The Retail Clerks' Association called for a 6 p.m. instead of a 9 p.m. closing on Saturdays to reduce staff exhaustion, but nothing was done until the employers' group—under pressure—made a similar request. *The Daily Province* reported that its carriers were affected, but promised to "carry to the last trench" to keep its readers up to date.

Fifteen city policemen were off sick. Forty postal workers were down. Many stores bore signs saying CLOSED BECAUSE OF FLU. The more than 100 beds moved into King Edward High School emergency hospital were now full.

At VGH, only one of the 40 nurses caring for flu victims was reported to have contracted the disease, and she had only a mild attack. St. Paul's hospital, however, was in a much worse state, with 10 nursing sisters (nuns) ill, along with 22 of 80 regular nurses.

George Ireland's sustained optimism began to fade as the situation deteriorated further. As hospital supplies ran out, he once again put out a call for donations of sheets and blankets. Volunteers were now urgently needed at all major hospitals to help replace sick laundry workers. The situation was compounded by a continuing strike at commercial laundry plants. One of the young women who responded to the call for volunteers was Mary Rogers, daughter of millionaire B.T. Rogers. She became ill, but survived.

South Vancouver was using an old school-board office as a temporary hospital. Abbotsford officials said they had no problems.

Ambulance drivers Joe Gibbs and Ed Slavin were working around the clock. The two came down with mild cases of the flu, but quickly returned to work because their services were so desperately needed. Driving could be dangerous. One newspaper report said a "delirious Italian" attacked an ambulance driver with a knife when he arrived to take the sick man to hospital.

The news from elsewhere offered little hope; all of it was ominous. Montreal and Toronto reported thousands dead. In Boston, one of the hardest-hit cities in the U.S., thousands were sick and many hundreds were dead and dying. Authorities said precautions were having little effect in halting the spread of the flu, although they hoped to hang on until the attack "burned itself out" as it appeared to have done in other places. Boston officials leaned heavily on the advantages of fresh air, advocating that, when possible, people be removed from their houses and regular hospitals and into tents where breezes could play on them. How this was to be tackled in cold winter temperatures wasn't explained.

Vancouver closes

On October 18, Fred Underhill finally gave in to local and provincial government pressure to cancel public gatherings and close all non-essential business services. He had felt from the beginning that many city closures across the country were merely cosmetic, meant to bolster politicians and persuade the populace that everything possible was being done, but he was anxious to keep the peace and get on with the job at hand. The doctor commented that the move would at least lift some of the responsibility from his shoulders, although he pointed out that nothing could stop people from stopping to talk or meeting at home with a group of friends. He felt the partial closure would make little difference. He believed the pandemic would continue until it eventually "burned out," as Boston medical specialists maintained.

His decision turned off the lights at schools, theatres, movie halls, poolrooms, dance pavilions, skating rinks, auction houses, churches, and exhibition halls. Club and union meetings were cancelled. Dr. Robert Wightman, the school-board doctor who had been in full agreement with Underhill's views about keeping the schools open and had conferred daily about the situation, now acquiesced with the move. The last day of operations for all of them was October 19.

That same evening the B.C. Coastal Steamship Service's *Princess Sophia* slipped out of Vancouver Harbour on a regularly scheduled voyage. She was heading up the coast for the round trip to Skagway,

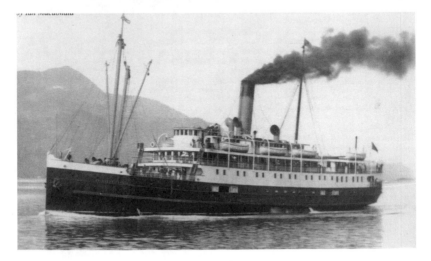

Those people who cancelled their trips on the Princess Sophia *due to the flu outbreak were the lucky ones, for the vessel met with disaster on her return trip from Skagway, Alaska.*

Alaska. There had been a couple of last-minute crew replacements because of the flu, and engineer Archie Alexander booked off the sailing because his twin baby daughters had come down with the disease and were ill in Victoria. The ailing crew members, Archie, and the girls would all survive, along with a crewman who missed the sailing because he stayed too long to say goodbye to his girlfriend.

It was one of the few instances of the flu working for good, for *Sophia* was embarking on her last voyage. It was the last major sailing of the year as winter took hold in the north. Rivers were icing up, and the men who manned the riverboats of the White Pass and Yukon Company were ready to head south, along with many other residents of Dawson City, Whitehorse, and communities across the Yukon Territories and Alaska. None of those who booked passage on the *Sophia*'s return leg from Skagway to Vancouver survived. Within a week, in one of the most tragic events in Canadian shipping history, the *Sophia* sank, making headlines of her own and greatly increasing the workload for gravediggers at Mountain View Cemetery in Vancouver.

LIVING WITH
THE SPANISH LADY

S ome of the strongest complaints about the Vancouver closures
came from church ministers who were unhappy with the
cancellation of services. They claimed their buildings were well
ventilated and that congregations needed a place to pray together in
these difficult times. Reverend W. Pascoe Goard made the point that
people were only in church once a week, for a relatively short time.
City hall, however, had made its decision and turned a deaf ear to
Goard's and all other objections.

The New Westminster police even got slightly over-zealous with
the closure order when they broke up an *outdoor* Salvation Army
service, which did not contravene the ban on indoor gatherings. When
the Sally-Ann raised objections, the constables agreed that it was
confusing, but said they didn't have any clear definitions on public
gatherings and were taking no chances.

Most shop owners and entertainment proprietors bore the
news stoically, knowing that objections would not sit well with a
public prepared to forgo its favourite outings in hopes of beating the
pandemic. Pool hall operators, though, apparently felt hard done by
and argued that their liberal use of disinfectants made their premises
completely safe and that they didn't accommodate crowds of people
at one time anyway. Unquestionably, some of the premises deemed
essential to the war effort were colder, draftier, less well ventilated,

and more congested than the blacked-out billiard parlours.

Entertainment was hard to come by. Libraries were closed, leaving residents with very little to occupy their leisure time. Library staff, still required to report to work, passed the time by catching up on cataloguing.

Vaudeville artists, actors, comedians, singers, and variety acts found themselves stranded. Theatres were closed up and down the whole west coast from Alaska to California, leaving many performers with no option but to sit out the pandemic wherever they happened to be. All they could do was hope that the curtain would rise again soon. In both Vancouver and Victoria, some entertainers gave free performances in hotel lobbies to practise their routines and to help pass the time.

Deprived of nights on the town, Vancouverites missed the antics of Charlie Chaplin and the emoting of Theda Bara in blood-and-thunder dramas. They didn't take kindly to one newspaper's suggestion that there were some advantages to being temporarily constrained to staying home at night. The idea of a "back to the songfest around the piano in the parlour" had no great appeal. Nevertheless, on the whole people took the situation "good naturedly and were prepared to put up with it."

Even the few businesses with permits to stay open did so under difficult conditions, often functioning with only about half of their normal number of employees. Fortunately, the number of customers was also down. B.C. Telephone Company reported that 83 of its operators were sick, and subscribers were asked to make phone calls only when absolutely necessary, as in this era before automation, each call had to be manually connected. Caterers and food distributors remained in operation but suffered from staff shortages, which sometimes resulted in late deliveries. Overall, the catering business suffered severe losses, as all large public functions were cancelled, and most families now preferred to eat at home rather than visit a restaurant.

Vancouver, barely into the third week of its fight against the pandemic, had nearly 900 confirmed flu cases, with 19 civilian and 13 military deaths. Two of the nurses from St. Paul's Hospital had joined the list of fatalities. Despite the flu's frightening escalation,

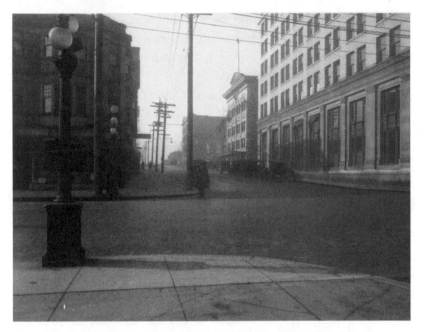

An eerie quiet envelops the deserted streets near the corner of Pender and Homer; along with other cities across the country, Vancouver eventually cancelled all public gatherings and closed all non-essential business services.

Underhill said that the city was fortunate in that its mortality rate was low compared to many other communities.

In outlying areas, there were far fewer cases than in cities. In the municipality of South Vancouver, an old school-board office was pressed into use as a temporary hospital, manned by a nurse and some volunteers. South Vancouver recorded its first death in the last week of October: streetcar conductor J. Goff, who died on the way to hospital. The mayor of South Vancouver was nursing his sick family at home when he received news of a second death, a baby on the Native reserve. Abbotsford officials reported having no problems at this point in time.

At about the same time, Richmond announced that it had 30 cases and had organized a careful watch on farm homes in the more remote areas of the Fraser River Delta. Reports from the rural Lower Mainland and many outlying areas of the province emphasized that more and more dwellings were being found where whole families were sick and barely able to cope with preparing food and keeping furnaces stoked. Neighbourhood volunteers were being organized to check regularly on isolated farms and to step in to help keep families alive wherever they were needed.

Vancouver's newspapers dubbed October 21 "Black Monday" although the highest daily death toll was yet to come. On the 21st, the number of dead stood at 33 and there were 1,300 people in hospital. Thirty-two nurses were off the job, and the King Edward High School emergency isolation centre, where the capacity had been increased to 200 beds, was full again.

The Victorian Order of Nurses appealed to people living near its Florence Nightingale Home to provide bed-and-breakfast accommodation for nurses who were working 12-hour shifts. This would save the women travelling time between the hospital and their residences and give them more rest.

Still the situation worsened, and the number of reported cases in Vancouver rose to 1,700. Close to 40 burials had taken place in the previous two days, underlining the need to find more gravediggers to cope with the increased number of funeral processions now arriving at the cemetery in a continuous stream. On October 25 Vancouver recorded 1,304 people in hospital. Two days later, on October 27, came the worst daily death toll so far: 24 people within 24 hours.

In Victoria, where the situation was no better, Dr. Price emphasized that reporting new cases was more important than ever. He said that some members of the Chinese community were caring for family members at home, and he felt they would be better tended to in hospitals.

Human cost and sacrifice

Fear of how many more would die was now a constant concern in Vancouver. The news across the continent was worse than ever and could no longer be ignored or brushed off. Vancouver was suffering like every other large city in North America, and still the Spanish Lady was claiming new victims.

In this era when religion played such a major role in everyday life, most people believed that catching the flu was a question of luck, and they seemed stoically resigned to the fact that pneumonia and death could follow. Many prayed nightly to be saved from the flu and trusted that God would take care of them. What baffled them most was the Spanish Lady's focus on 20- to 40-year-olds. Nothing like it had ever been seen before anywhere. Surely the young men of the country were suffering enough in the war. More deaths were unthinkable ... yet the daily toll continued.

A young policeman with five years on the force, Constable McGillivray (No. 205), was listed as a victim. The Vancouver business world was saddened by the death of Charles "Bill" Hartley, a man of only 32 who in a short time had built up a booming wholesale business from a small cigar store on Hastings Street. He left behind a widow and two small children. The same day, a 19-year-old student nurse, Irene Jones, died at St. Paul's Hospital after caring for the sick for days without sufficient rest.

The Vancouver Daily Sun paid special tribute to a young doctor who had sacrificed his own life, 31-year-old W.C. Swenerton, described as one of Vancouver's more promising young surgeons. He had worked himself to exhaustion, taken a few days off, and then returned to work. Flu struck him suddenly, as it often did, and he died a day later after suffering the symptoms of pneumonia. He left behind a wife, who was down with the flu, and two young children.

One man who recovered paid tribute to the care and treatment he received while in hospital. L.W. Carlew said he had received wonderful care, despite the tremendous load being carried by doctors, nurses, and all those involved in keeping hospitals running.

The pressing city-wide shortage of clean laundry was finally alleviated by a strike-ending agreement with the commercial cleaners. Laundries were considered essential services, and the lack of them during the early weeks of the pandemic had hampered families and institutions alike. Female workers were happy to learn they would now be paid $12 to $18 a week; men would receive $22 to $25. Drivers were to get salary plus commission, and the new contract stated that women could now apply to be classified as drivers—a breakthrough for them.

Ever-overworked relief organizer George Ireland said his latest appeal for help had brought in 50 volunteer nurses; half of them were immediately sent to private residences where they were urgently needed. They included "young ladies prominent in society," he said. He paid particular tribute to some teenagers who had offered their services but had to be turned down because they were considered too young. Older men were still needed for the heavier lifting and carrying at hospitals. Ireland was not satisfied with the response he had so far received and sharply criticized the small number of volunteers coming forward to fill the gaps in the medical workforce. "We are wringing our hands and unable to help, in many cases because women of the city who are in a position to assist as a duty are not doing so," an irate Ireland told *The Daily Province*. "All we can do is appeal to the consciences of these ladies who can give us assistance but have not done so." He zeroed in on recently idled schoolteachers who were not coming forward "in appropriate numbers" to help now that the schools were closed. At the same time he thanked those who *had* come forward and were serving in makeshift isolation wards.

Fear of catching the flu and dying was the stumbling block. Many people were not prepared to risk their own lives by getting too close to strangers who were seriously ill. The escalating shortage of helpers produced a radical suggestion for the times when civic officials recommended that men also be used as volunteer nurses. It didn't happen.

Members of the Independent Order Daughters of the Empire had organized and were now operating a soup kitchen at Aberdeen School. They put out a call to the public, seeking containers for soups and stews for delivery to homes where family members were too sick to cook for themselves.

Ireland's pleading and chastising comments finally did bring better results, providing 70 additional volunteers, although more were needed. He had had calls for help from 32 more families unable to cope on their own. In addition, he said, people continued to arrive daily in boats from up-coast and were being taken to St. Paul's Hospital, the closest facility to the city docks. Unfortunately, St. Paul's now had more sick nurses than VGH or St. Mary's in New Westminster. Superintendent McPhillips had also taken to his bed for a week but had returned to work. Ireland said the city likely was looking at a $50,000 bill for its relief operations.

Doctors throughout the city repeated their warnings to people to keep their feet dry. The warnings this time were prompted by a heavy downpour, again hailed by Dr. Underhill as a godsend to wash away germ-laden dust and smoke.

Of course, not everyone was sick, and some of the cheeriest people in town could be seen in lineups of 100 or more at the government liquor outlet on Beattie Street. Wartime prohibition banned liquor sales, but with a doctor's certificate and a $2 permit, those in need could obtain a bottle of their choosing. Obliging doctors cited such things as flu prevention and stress relief as reasons for "prescribing" liquor for the grinning folk who waited in line for the medicine they wanted.

In Victoria the lines were just as long as those in Vancouver, as men happily waited their turn outside the capital's official liquor outlet. Prohibition Commissioner W.C. Findlay said that despite sharp increases in the number of so-called ailing, there was enough liquor to "meet all legitimate needs." Findlay later made headlines when he was charged with stealing 74 cases for his own use.

News coverage was still less than complete in patriotic Vancouver, which to a large extent remained focused on the war in Europe. During the early stages of the pandemic, the two main Vancouver newspapers had been reluctant to run flu stories on their front pages. Now that the pandemic was a major crisis throughout the province, ravaging all of Canada and the world, the *Sun* was giving the disease front-page coverage. However, it was hard to comprehend why the flu still received little attention from the *Province*, other than a mention on page five or six.

At the end of October the *Sun* ran one odd little item that presumably was intended as a light-hearted exhortation in the midst of a lot of bad news. It said: "Cheer up, Good morning, The flu is on the wane, Don't worry, Attend to business, Shop as Usual, Doing Nicely Thank You, Now Altogether, Smile, smile, smile." Unfortunately, the editors were wrong. That same day Dr. Underhill announced the month-end totals for the flu. The city had treated 1,844 cases and recorded about 170 deaths. The pandemic was far from over.

Through it all there was little criticism of the policies or performance of politicians, medical authorities, or health workers.

There were a few citizens who contended they hadn't been told enough, but Underhill answered their criticism by explaining that there wasn't a budget for mounting a massive information campaign. He pointed to the good job the papers had done in informing the public, even though their coverage wasn't front-page news. Perhaps this was why some readers had missed his earlier comments and suggestions and felt ill informed.

There was little to boost morale in reports emanating from across Canada or anywhere in the world. In some cities the pandemic seemed to be abating, but in other locations the number of cases continued to climb. Toronto had 76 deaths in one day; Bombay had 768 deaths over a week; Paris recorded almost 900 new cases in 24 hours. It seemed to make little difference whether cities had shut down most of their public places or left them in full operation; the Spanish Lady struck with the same ferocity.

Death was everywhere in 1918. It was almost impossible to avoid daily news of lives lost or threatened either by the war or the pandemic.

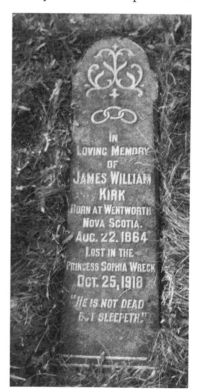

Beside and among the graves of those who died of the flu are those of travellers from the north who perished in the sinking of the Canadian Pacific ship Princess Sophia.

The wife of Corporal T.G. Wood was a typical case. She received one of the dreaded wires that arrived in Vancouver with great regularity. Her husband wasn't dead, but he had been wounded in the head, face, and arm. It was the third such wire she had received. The soldier had been in France for three years, and previously he had been gassed and wounded. She fervently hoped that this time he would be sent home—and that he wouldn't contract the flu.

People grasped at straws, and stories or rumours of new cures surfaced in a steady stream. In Chicago, doctors angrily denounced the claims of a fellow physician who contended that diphtheria serum could cure the flu. One newly suggested remedy, almost certain to ward off most humans, was rubbing the chest with a mixture of goose grease and turpentine. Dr. Underhill, always the voice of reason, told residents not to build up their hopes, as he knew of no new developments for an effective safeguard, medicine, treatment, or vaccine.

One encouraging note about the war was contained in a letter that a young Vancouver soldier, Private Alfred John Levy, wrote to his parents. He had worked as a newspaperman in Prince Rupert and New Westminster before joining up. He wrote that he believed the more bloodthirsty generals had finally stopped launching futile attacks that killed thousands and spoke of a new offensive that might lead to war's end.

"We could plainly see that there are real brains behind us and it was no fool's errand we were on," Levy wrote from the front. He described how tanks were crushing enemy machine-gun posts, Allied planes were dropping bombs, kilted pipers were leading attacks, and cavalry units were rounding up enemy prisoners. Sadly, this new initiative did nothing for young Levy, who was killed in action shortly after writing his letter.

Vancouver, Victoria, and Seattle, all reeling from the ravages of war and the pandemic, were now struck with another disaster. Many people were so numbed that it was impossible for them to take in the details of the latest huge death toll. On Sunday, October 27, they learned the fate of the Canadian Pacific Coastal steamer *Princess Sophia*. Eight days earlier she had set out from Vancouver's Pier D. The six-year-old coastal liner, built particularly for the Vancouver–Victoria–Seattle run to Alaska, had run aground on Vanderbilt Reef just four hours after leaving Skagway on her return voyage south. The ship remained hard aground on the rock for 40 hours before 65-year-old Captain Leonard Locke, his crew, and everyone aboard—an estimated 360 people—went to their deaths in the icy waters of Lynn Canal during a violent snowstorm on October 25. The dead included men, women, children, horses, and pets. The only survivor was a black dog. Because telegraph lines had been down, it had taken nearly two days for the news to reach the outside world.

When the ill-fated vessel had arrived in Skagway to load passengers and their baggage on October 23, Captain Locke had hired 10 temporary crewmen because six regulars were down with the flu and could not work. The afflicted crewmen could not be sent to hospital ashore because the Alaska governor had placed a ban on anyone with flu setting foot in his state. The sick seamen stayed aboard and died there, along with their replacements and a number of additional passengers who had wormed their way aboard. *Princess Sophia* was carrying an extra 50 passengers when she sank.

In the first few days after the tragedy many bodies were recovered. They were taken to Juneau, Alaska, to await the arrival of another Canadian Pacific coastal liner, the *Princess Alice*, which would take them home for burial in Vancouver, Victoria, Seattle, and other U.S. destinations. When the *Alice* arrived in Juneau, Alaska regulations again prevented the crew from disembarking, and bodies were loaded aboard from a barge that was towed out into the harbour. Because of her tragic cargo, *Princess Alice* became known as "the ship of sorrow."

The *Alice* sailed for Vancouver carrying 159 bodies recovered from the sea, six of them unidentified. The hunt for the remaining bodies would continue for nearly a year. Pier D in Vancouver was draped in black for her arrival, even though she docked at 11 p.m. It was the day the Armistice was signed, November 11, 1918, and elsewhere the city was bright with lights and banners brought out for the celebrations. Bonfires burned on high points around the city and residents partied into the night, except for those who waited at Pier D to identify the bodies of loved ones. The graves of those who had died from the flu and from the wreck of the *Princess Sophia* lie in adjacent areas in Vancouver's Mountain View Cemetery.

Two Vancouver families were thankful that they had escaped the fatal final voyage of the steamer, but they were only briefly saved from sorrow. Crewman Joseph Woosman contracted the flu during *Sophia's* journey north and was taken to hospital in Prince Rupert. He escaped the awful wreck at Vanderbilt Reef, but flu claimed him only a few days later in hospital. He left a wife and a child in Vancouver. Passenger J. Austin Fraser had also counted himself lucky because he had cancelled his sailing on the *Sophia* only an hour before she embarked from Vancouver, but while visiting Seattle in early November he, too, died of flu.

Governor Thomas Riggs Jr.'s ban on travel into Alaska was a major factor in delaying the Spanish Lady's arrival in Dawson City, Yukon. The strict quarantines he imposed were of considerable help to Canadians living in this northern outpost. He banned all travel from Alaskan communities into Canada and even halted mail delivery for the winter season. As a result, it was April 1919 before the pandemic reached Dawson, and by then it was a much less severe strain than had ravaged Alaska in the fall.

The debate over masks

As the pandemic raged on and the number of deaths continued to rise across North America, some medical authorities ordered that masks be worn in public, often imposing penalties if the regulation was not obeyed. In Calgary, where masks were mandatory, 100 residents were fined for failing to wear them. In B.C., debate arose once again, partly because Underhill and Price held differing views on the subject.

Victoria's Price was against the wearing masks under any circumstances. He contended that they only collected germs and did not help prevent the flu from spreading. Underhill wasn't prepared to suggest they be mandatory in Vancouver, but he did recommend that managers of banks, stores, and similar essential operations—those still dealing with the public—encourage their staff to wear them. Underhill very much believed in preserving the freedom of the individual to make his or her own decision. He felt that if he explained why he had made a recommendation, the people of Vancouver would do the right thing for themselves and the rest of the community.

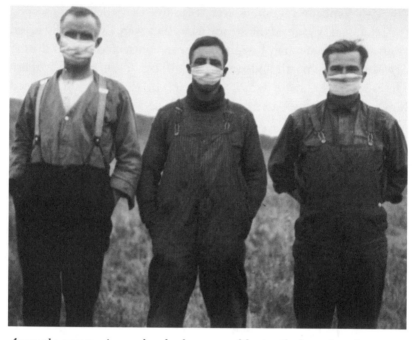

Across the country, in rural and urban areas alike, people donned masks to protect themselves against the flu. The practice of wearing surgical masks was hotly debated in the medical community.

Masks and tight-fitting veils became so common on city streets that a Vancouver *Daily Province* reporter wrote, "The ravishing Houri of the mystic east peeping shyly above the fragrant webbing of the nose veil protecting all features from the common gaze of the infidel has nothing on the Vancouver girls whose facial contours are hidden by the new flu veils." The reporter feared that some girls were wearing the veils too tightly and might have trouble breathing.

Dr. Underhill pointed out that veils, masks, and the variety of scarves being worn to cover noses and mouths needed to be changed frequently if they were to serve the purpose for which they were intended. He encouraged barbers and dentists to follow Seattle's example and wear masks at all times when shaving customers or pulling teeth. The situation was critical in Washington State; the population was dealing with high levels of fear and depression. Some store owners in Seattle threatened to refuse service to anyone not wearing a mask.

Authorities across Canada were either recommending or mandating masks and, in some cases, describing how to construct them. Needless to say, some businesses leapt into the breach. Vancouver's Tom the Tailor advertised what he claimed was the perfect flu preventative: a partial face mask that he was selling for 35 cents each or $3.50 a dozen. He proclaimed that the mask was cool to wear and made of pure wool, with a medicated camphor interior. Drawings showed how it looked. "You fear no grippe when you are wearing one of these," Tom contended. Described as "Vancouver's very own invention," each mask contained a layer of all-wool broadcloth, in either black or white, lined with sateen "with a pocket in between treated with a disinfectant chemical preparation." When a mask was washed, the disinfectant could be replaced, claimed Tom, adding that they were selling in the hundreds. Most knew the preventative claim was questionable, but soon even the wariest people were wearing them on the streets.

Medical opinion was split on the question of masks throughout the pandemic. Some doctors complained that those made of cheesecloth quickly became dirty, wet, and clammy and that an all-wool mask like Tom's was a major improvement. Others insisted that masks did little to prevent catching the flu. Dr. Underhill chose not to comment on this particular issue.

As the situation become more critical, organizations throughout the city did what they could to help. The Rotary Club organized a volunteer taxi service among its members to ferry doctors, nurses, and clergy to the now full emergency hospital at King Edward High School. Hill Tire Company offered free repairs to all cars being used in the shuttle service.

Belatedly, the Canadian Pacific Railway announced from its Vancouver headquarters that it was fumigating all railway cars and advised the public not to travel unless it was absolutely necessary. Had this step been taken earlier, it might have helped thwart the Spanish Lady's intentions.

Within only a few days, she had claimed another 27 victims. Among them were nursing sister Syncletique and nurse Eulalia Lanovite, both from St. Paul's hospital in Vancouver. Nurse Kathleen Bryant was also hailed as a heroine for her unswerving service day and night to the sick at St. Paul's. Unable to continue one night because she was ill, she

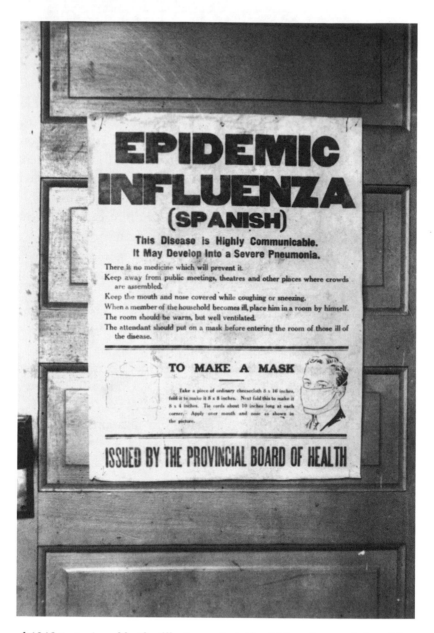

A 1918 poster issued by the Alberta provincial health board warned the public about the Spanish flu and offered instructions for making protective masks.

insisted on going home rather than occupying a hospital bed. She never returned to her duties.

Miss Ruth Luno died at VGH. She was a schoolteacher who had taught in Burnaby and then at Lord Nelson School. When Underhill ordered its closure, she had answered one of Ireland's early pleas for help and volunteered to work in the hospital. She had already brought her mother and sister back to health at home. Unfortunately, she was not one of the lucky ones: She died only two weeks after joining the volunteer staff. Today, a plaque honouring Ruth B. Luno, Pearl Alberta Green, and Alice Ross Rines—"teachers who gave their lives for others"—hangs in the hallway of Lord Nelson School. When the plaque was dedicated in mid-1919, teacher G.I. Ward and Livingstone School principal R.F. Caldwell were also named as deserving of honour.

Despite the fear and trauma of the time, the crisis contained the odd humorous situation. A doctor hurried to a South Vancouver home in answer to a call from a man who had suddenly taken ill. The harried practitioner arrived to find the man in bed, fully clothed and wearing

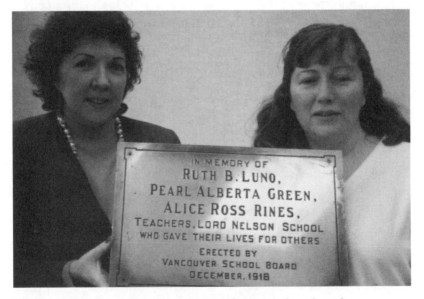

Teachers were among those who volunteered to nurse the sick, and some gave their lives in the fight. Lord Nelson School Principal Nicole Boucher, left, and school librarian Janet Lirenman hold up a plaque, recently rediscovered and remounted, that was put up at the school to honour three of them.

dirty workboots. When he was asked what his complaint was, the man said he had remembered reading that when symptoms appeared it was advisable to go straight to bed. He had been working in his garden when he felt "shooting pains," so he took the recommended action. He rushed into the house and jumped into bed, clothes, boots, and all. His pains had abated by the time the doctor arrived, and he was diagnosed as flu-free.

Crisis becomes desperate

With the number of deaths rising, and sickness escalating among the army of volunteers, it became more difficult than ever to handle the daily workload. During one shift at Royal Columbian Hospital in New Westminster, only one superintendent and two regular staff nurses were able to work. In an era when few married women worked, the hospital was supported almost totally by married graduate nurses from the area who had volunteered to return to duty during the pandemic. Kitchens and the hospital's other services were being maintained by volunteers. Army nursing sister Marjorie Beatrice Moberley became the first military nurse to die at nearby Coquitlam's hospital.

Vancouver Mayor Gale reiterated Ireland's call for more volunteers, using even stronger language and an angrier tone, hoping it would jolt the consciences of those who had failed to respond. In a front-page story in both newspapers, Gale said a severe shortage of nurses was adding greatly to Vancouver's problems. He insisted the situation at city hospitals must not be allowed to continue and demanded a response from all people in homes unaffected by the pandemic.

"People are actually dying in considerable numbers without the care and attention that even the meanest stranger within our gates is entitled to," Gale charged. He said hospital staffs were worn out to the stage where they sometimes were unable to provide what was needed. "Do those who could give assistance realize how greatly their services are required? This appeal is to every man and woman who can possibly volunteer to do their bit."

The mayor again made pointed comments about those dowagers who employed privately hired nurses to look after other ailments and demanded that they "release them for the larger need that is so urgent." Passionately, he expounded: "Medical staffs are working to the point of exhaustion, battling night and day with hardly time to catch a morsel of food, and scarcely a chance to get a wink of sleep. The brave little band of trained nurses and volunteer assistants tackling the epidemic at VGH have issued a cry for help through Dr. McEachern, the medical superintendent who said many were working double shifts. Will you offer your services to save lives?"

The situation by early November was indeed desperate, and Gale's final comments confirmed that hospitals would take anyone who came forward. He emphasized that no nursing experience was needed and that volunteers would tend only to non-contagious patients. Exactly how this would be possible was not explained, but Gale wanted help and felt he might get it by playing down the fear factor, which in the early days of November had become more evident.

Men were also needed to do heavy work, and teenaged boys were sought to carry meals from the kitchens to the wards. The volunteers would work eight-hour shifts, either from 8 a.m. to 4 p.m., from 4 to midnight, or from 12 a.m. to 8 a.m. Gale emphasized that the worst was far from over. The severe staff shortage had brought a request from the hospitals for the public to stop sending flowers to relatives and loved ones because there was no one to put them in vases or water them.

The mayor said later that the response to his impassioned call to arms had been good; he had obviously hit a responsive chord in the hearts of Vancouverites by bringing the stark reality of the situation, the life-and-death drama being enacted in his city, to their attention. Several dozen new volunteers had stepped forward. Typical was the offer by a woman to work nights after her husband came home from his job and could look after the children. Ireland reported that he had 100 families listed who required help and was better able to send assistance to them because of the mayor's call. At this point, he too succumbed to the flu, but suffered only a mild attack and was back on the job within a few days.

Among the newly volunteered was a woman from Victoria, Agnes Jean Chambers, who tended the Nunley family until the father died and then stayed on to care for his widow and children. Within days she too became a victim of the flu and quickly died.

Occasionally the newspapers, as a possible inducement for volunteers to come forward, ran the names of the latest residents willing to offer their services. They also listed contributions that had been made to help the sick, ranging from tobacco from the Hudson's Bay Company to two boxes of apples from a Mr. Teaf.

The emergency unit at King Edward reminded relatives and friends of patients that they were not permitted to visit and that they need not bring meals for their loved ones, as these were being supplied from the school cafeteria. Police chief William McRae asked motorists to avoid the area around the school-cum-hospital in order to keep it clear for the ambulance service. Between them, the main hospital and the isolation centre had now admitted a total of 2,387 patients.

The gravity of the pandemic was driven home further by newspaper reports that Montreal's death toll was now up to 2,258. Vancouver by this time had treated 3,092 cases and listed more than 200 dead. Burnaby, affected little by the flu at the start of the outbreak, now had 28 cases, and a fireman was the municipality's first fatality. Charles Hern, a CPR section foreman, was suburban Maple Ridge's first death.

Statistics from the United States were even more staggering. As many as 211,000 cases were reported by November in army camps throughout the country, and there were 7,132 deaths. Only a few days later these totals had risen to 250,000 cases and 10,741 deaths.

As the pandemic peaked, the problems multiplied. More and more families were being found where all members were sick in bed at home and barely able to care for each other. Isolated pockets of people in distress were also being discovered. Several critically ill and dying men, who had been laying rail line in an isolated area of the Fraser Valley, were found and brought to Vancouver with the hope that VGH could save their lives. Not far away in the Fraser Delta, thousands of tons of potatoes were rotting in the fields because there was nobody to harvest them. The list of cancelled celebrations such as weddings also grew longer.

Vancouverites often recognized prominent people among the flu victims named in the news. Prominent shipping man Captain Robert Turner was rushed by special ferry from his home on Bowen Island but died within hours of being admitted to St. Paul's. Abroad,

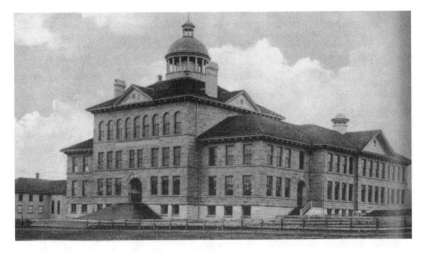

Across the province and the country, schools such as King Edward High School in Vancouver, pictured here, were pressed into service as emergency flu hospitals.

the most recent victims included the son of writer Sir Arthur Conan Doyle, Dr. Conan Doyle, who died in England, and Prince Eric in Sweden. Future U.S. president Franklin D. Roosevelt caught the flu but survived, as did England's King George V.

First signs of hope

Finally in Vancouver there was reduced pressure on the ambulance service, and Dr. Underhill saw hope in the fact that the number of patients being discharged daily from VGH was growing. This took some of the pressure off him and his overworked, bone-weary staff. St. Paul's and other hospitals in the Lower Mainland also were carrying lighter loads. In South Vancouver, where Selkirk School had been converted into an emergency isolation centre, the teachers, janitors, and maintenance employees who stepped in to care for patients were praised for their "noble work."

As signs appeared indicating the pandemic might ebb, the stoic, unflappable but tiring Dr. Underhill himself fell ill. He continued to work after suffering the first symptoms, something he had told the public not to do, but was worn down and eventually had to take to his bed. He stubbornly refused to occupy scarce hospital space, and

127

was nursed by Beatrice and other members of the family.

From his sickbed, Underhill demanded regular daily reports on how the city was faring and gave orders as he saw fit. He also took the opportunity to call for extra compensation for health workers who had toiled mightily since the flu had struck, but the city fathers didn't rush to agree. It would be "considered," they said. The flu outbreak had already cost Vancouver an estimated $36,000, and council agreed to make an additional $17,000 payment to VGH.

In Victoria, provincial officials announced that B.C. was losing $500 a day in taxes because of the entertainment-site closures, but the increasing sale of liquor for "medicinal purposes" was helping.

Vancouverites again ignored warnings about spreading the disease when they crowded downtown for another Victory Loan drive. They cheered as Harry Gardiner, "The Human Fly," dressed all in white, scaled the walls of the Hotel Vancouver to unfurl a banner. Officials raised no objections to the performance, but when Gardiner appeared days later in Victoria, Dr. Price dashed off a blistering letter to the *Victoria Colonist* in which he made it abundantly clear that the man's performance was held against his recommendation. With entertainment centres shut, boredom had set in and a sizeable crowd had gathered on the street to watch the daredevil climb a downtown building. Price wrote angrily, "People seem to be not aroused to the danger of flu. I might have to impose tougher restrictions." He slammed the organizer of the event for promoting a silly sideshow and said it was a foolhardy and useless stunt in which a man endangered himself and the spectators endangered themselves. He added that the pandemic was a war in the midst of Victoria. "Don't sneer at the enemy," he said, "because the undertakers are waiting."

This Victory Loan drive was keyed to the end of hostilities in Europe, but there remained stark reminders that neither fighting nor pandemic was over yet. Two Vancouver policemen, privates William Morrison and James Watson, were both killed on the same day at the front. They had joined the medical corps together as stretcher bearers. *The Province* told its readers that Watson fell while taking part in a gallant charge. Morrison recovered his body and brought it back to Canadian lines, but a few hours later death came to him "in the same way boldly fighting the enemies of civilization and humanity." Ill health prevented Lieutenant Charles Duncan, 31, of the Tenth New Westminster Regiment from going overseas: He joined the casualty lists as a victim of the flu. George Blackman had survived the carnage of the assault and the victory by Canadians at Vimy Ridge, although it had cost him a leg, but he couldn't beat the disease. He died at home in Vancouver, leaving behind a young widow and son.

Businesses in Victoria were now complaining bitterly about loss of revenue and the continued ban on places of recreation. Members of the Merchants Association, noticing signs that the pandemic might be on the way out, made a special appeal to Price, but he adamantly refused to change his position. One small-business operator said he was losing $150 a day. Poolroom proprietor Jack O'Brien claimed he had lost $2,500 since the ban began. He maintained that he was one of the heaviest losers and blasted Price and his policy. Reverend William Stevenson added his voice to the appeal, saying it was unworthy to close churches and it should be remembered that religion was medicine for the soul. Price wouldn't budge.

As the gloomy, wet November wore on, the weary population of British Columbia tried to cope with more hardship, sorrow, and

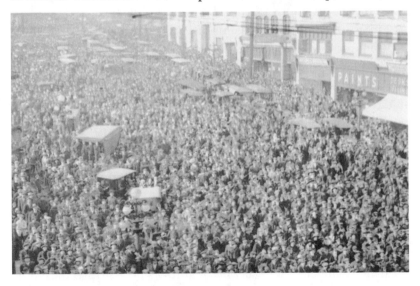

Crowds on Beatty Street in Vancouver, ignoring dire warnings about public gatherings, came out in full force for a Victory Loan drive and cheered on Harry Gardiner, "The Human Fly.

disease than seemed humanly possible. "Germany on the Way Out for Sure" was the headline in *The Daily Province*, but Vancouverites had read similar optimistic reports before. They were living through the greatest and most horrible military war in history, and it was dragging into its fifth year. Their local battle with the Spanish flu was only a month old, but it too seemed to have been going on forever. Despite the hopeful signs, as one patient recovered, another one fell ill. Every day there was a new crisis.

The gravedigger shortage became even more acute. Thought was given to moving steam shovels into the graveyard in order to alleviate the problem, but in an era when religion played a significant role in daily life, this suggestion appalled the vast majority of people. The idea was dismissed, and somehow enough men and boys with shovels were found to provide graves for another 25 bodies, which had arrived from the isolated Britannia Copper Smelter on Howe Sound. Accessible only by sea, the community of Britannia had already shipped more than 100 sick and dying flu victims to Vancouver.

Mayor Gale petitioned Dr. Young in Victoria to permit 6 p.m. store closings in order to take some of the strain off hard-pressed grocery and drugstore clerks, who were doing their best to serve customers under difficult circumstances. Tempers often flared when the lines for food and other essentials were long.

Few outlets did not have a number of employees off sick, and those workers still on their feet were nearing exhaustion. Ernest Rea, secretary of the Vancouver branch of the Retail Clerks' Protective Association, was one of many who wrote to the mayor asking for reduced hours on Saturday to give shop clerks a longer weekend to rest. Many were working from 8 a.m. to 10 p.m., a 14-hour day broken only by short periods when they took time out to eat the lunch and dinner sandwiches they had brought with them. H.E. Wills, manager of Economy Meat, also wrote to the mayor asking for reduced hours, but noted: "I sincerely hope that all Greek and Chinese are included as that is only fair to our white employees." Wills was expressing the prejudices of the day, referring to the fact that many meat stores catering to specific ethnic groups were open longer hours and sold meat cheaper than the regular butchers, whose clientele included the majority white population. The government agreed to the request for early store closings, but only after the clerks received support in writing from the Retail Merchants Association, which represented the employers. This early closing applied only to essential-services outlets such as food and pharmacy operations, which remained open during the pandemic.

Store owners suffering through the total closure began to complain more loudly. Cigar-store operators said they were being treated unfairly, since drugstores, which were excluded from the closing order, also sold tobacco products and were getting an unfair advantage. Vancouver Tobacco Company Limited went so far as to maintain that their products were medicines that helped tackle flu, and so should be readily available. Their plea went unanswered.

At this point Dr. Edwin D. Carder, the acting assistant medical health officer, offered another ray of hope. Filling in for the afflicted Dr. Underhill, he announced a reduction in the number of new cases. However, there was disturbing news that after more than a week in bed, the man in charge of fighting the flu in Vancouver was in a weakened condition. Underhill was now fighting off the Spanish Lady's attentions directly. One of his daughters, Helen, had also contracted the disease while working as a volunteer nurse and was said to be quite sick. Another daughter, Enid, laboured on as a volunteer, while Beatrice Underhill continued to minister to her ailing family at home.

THE PANDEMIC BURNS OUT

L ocal hospitals were now coping more efficiently than they had a month earlier. Time had given supervisory staff the opportunity to reorganize shifts and duties so that no one was required to work the long hours that had been in effect through October. As the pandemic continued, greater cooperation developed among municipalities, and officials were able to eliminate duplication and waste of services. Various labour organizations stepped in and helped to set up a centralized temporary employment system for all of Greater Vancouver.

There was more good news. Dr. Underhill had not joined the ranks of the flu's victims and was able to return to work. The recovery of other family members, as well, testified to the efficacy of his methods and the nursing capabilities of Beatrice.

Meanwhile, the search went on in laboratories throughout the world for a cure. In Spain, a Dr. Maldone was said to have isolated microbes he claimed were responsible for the Spanish flu. Maldone said it was not bacillus Pfeiffer, "but one approaching in character to that of the bubonic plague." Medical opinion was divided, although some experts thought it might explain why the Spanish flu struck so quickly and could kill within hours. Yet another report stated that vaccines seemed to work in some cases but definitely not in all.

Newspapers printed every new, supposed cure for a population that had become desperate, and Underhill felt it necessary to tell Vancouverites that nothing effective was being manufactured locally. At

133

home, publicity-seeking Dr. Robert A. McKay was offering to swallow flu germs from patients every day for a week in order to back up his contention that germs and microbes were not causing the sickness. He claimed that many medical men agreed with him. He maintained that flu was spread by people sitting in stuffy offices and on drafty streetcars with open windows. The only protection, he contended, was warm clothing, combined with avoiding drafts and exposure to cold. Nobody took him up on his offer to swallow germs.

Public places remained closed, and the lack of services and everyday comforts was beginning to pall on everyone; as a result, people began to find ways of getting around any regulations they considered inappropriate. St. George's Anglican Church and the First Baptist Church in Vancouver held outdoor Sunday services, which were well attended. And, unlike the earlier episode with the Salvation Army, the authorities didn't find the downtown churches in violation of regulations.

Going a little further, Reverend F.E. Farris of St. John's Anglican Church in North Vancouver reopened his church and was totally unrepentant when he was fined $10 for conducting a Sunday service. He told the court that by permitting stores, offices, and factories to remain open, but not churches, the "law is serving Mammon instead of God." Two token members of his congregation were fined $2.50 each for attending the service. But maybe their prayers helped: A newspaper headline noted that with a continuing drop in the number of cases, the flu situation was "encouraging."

It was initially an illusory hope. The pattern was the same across Canada and around the world: The situation would seem to improve, then slip back, then improve again. When the case level seemed to be dropping in Vancouver and there was talk of closing the King Edward emergency unit, it suddenly soared again. When physicians in Winnipeg believed the worst was over, hundreds of new cases and deaths were suddenly reported. In England and Wales the death toll was terrible, approaching 32,000 people in a six-week period.

VGH's Dr. McEachern, who earlier had been optimistic that the flu was on the way out, said he would have to review the entire situation. Many new cases, including a sudden 75 at the industrial school at Point Grey, plus 15 more deaths, gave him cause for reconsidering. Officials at King Edward emergency hospital made another pitch for donations of linen, particularly pieces 18 by 15 inches for making poultices.

Two suicides were reported, of men said to be delirious with the flu. One shot himself, and the other was killed when he jumped off a veranda at the Oakalla jail in Burnaby.

The city's finest young men continued to fall before the Spanish Lady. Dr. J. F. McNeill, 35, the priest at the city's Sacred Heart Church, died at St. Paul's. He had answered every call to the hospital to minister to the sick and dying and was praised for never sparing himself. Constable Brundige, 30, became the third policeman to die, leaving a widow and two small children. Constable George Clerke, the fourth policeman to die, was described as a man of "splendid physique and wonderful vitality and one of the department's best athletes." He left a widow and child.

Thirty-year-old Ian Grant Forbes, a former Vancouver bank employee who headed east to train as a flier, got no farther than Toronto. He died of flu at a military base there three months after he had joined up. A New Westminster soccer star, Jimmy Craig of the Royal City Rovers, was also a victim. J. R. Robertson, a prominent B.C. athlete and member of Vancouver's Celtic Soccer Club, was luckier. He survived fierce trench fighting as a lieutenant in the army and was awarded the Croix de Guerre for bravery by the French government, and he also escaped the flu.

In November, all nine members of the Blatchford family were sick at their Huntington farm home in the Fraser Valley. Despite running a temperature at times well over 102 degrees Fahrenheit, the patriarch struggled outside to milk his cows and, with the help of neighbours, kept his farm going.

As a break from sad and depressing news, there finally were real indications that people could expect the end of the war. On November 6 *The Vancouver Daily Sun* proudly told its readers that it had arranged with the B.C. Electric Company to help inform people the moment it happened. Announcing an end to one of the tragedies besetting the world was a project every newspaper publisher wanted to be in on. There were few radios at this time, and word could only be spread by telephone or by the pealing of bells and the tooting of sirens.

To signify the end of hostilities, BCE would trigger mechanisms that would make house and office lights all over the city flicker three times. Of course, this wouldn't make much difference to people in bed with the lights out, but the paper trumpeted the scheme.

Early the next morning, on November 7, the bells pealed, the sirens screamed, and people rushed out into the streets cheering and hugging their neighbours. Lights started coming on all over town. Some business operations immediately announced there would be a half-day holiday, but it was all a false alarm. The joy faded fast as the disappointing word spread. A wire report from Europe had been misinterpreted; the guns were still booming. Tears streamed from many eyes when it was realized that hopes had been dashed once again.

In the early hours of November 11, the population finally learned that the war was truly over. Ships in the harbour blew their whistles in harmony with factory sirens and church bells. This time, an armistice had been signed in France. Soon there were large singing and cheering crowds everywhere. Impromptu parades wound through the streets, accompanied by the banging of saucepans, the wail of bagpipes, and the blare of a bugle or two. Street dances erupted spontaneously at downtown intersections, and congregations flocked to special church services to give thanks. Celebrations continued all day and well into the night, as residents delved into cabinets where a supply of liquor had been kept for medicinal purposes. Bonfires blazed on the beaches and on the hillsides surrounding Vancouver harbour. For a little while the flu was forgotten.

In marked contrast to the end-of-war celebrations, funeral corteges continued to wend their way through the streets. A Vancouver doctor, an obstetrician named John Barker, later recalled, "I was still in bed when the Armistice was signed. I remember the funerals passing along Sixth Avenue that same day. Nurses were almost unobtainable and doctors were so overworked that during the time I was ill, I had five different doctors. They worked themselves into a state of exhaustion, but returned as soon as possible when another one dropped. It was terrible. Many of my friends died."

Only a few paid heed as the darkened *Princess Alice*, "the ship of sorrow," sailed slowly through the narrows off Stanley Park that

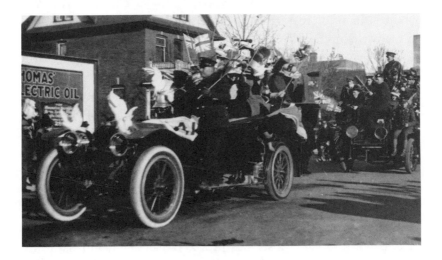

Even at the victory parades that took place across the country on November 11, 1918, participants wore protective masks.

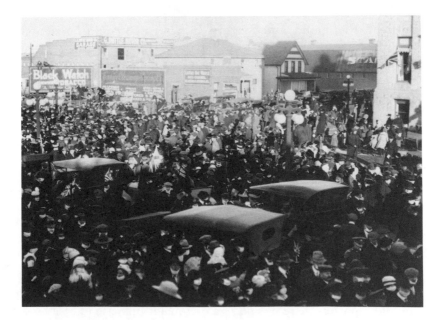

night and made her berth on the waterfront, where the bodies of passengers from the *Sophia* were laid out for identification. The *Alice* later continued on to Victoria and Seattle. The Puget Sound city had so many victims both from the flu and from the shipwreck in Alaska that the mayor sent a message to Vancouver requesting all the flowers that could be spared for funeral wreaths.

November 11, 1918, was a momentous day around the world, even for the flu. In the mid-Atlantic a drama took place when most of the crew of a ship sailing from Montevideo, Uruguay, to Europe fell ill, and passengers who hadn't succumbed took their places to bring the vessel into port.

The next day a Vancouver newspaper headline read: "Flu Reduced To Very Small Figures"—more a result of the optimism and the exuberance of the armistice celebrations than anything else. Underhill feared a serious problem remained, and, sadly, he was proven correct when the pendulum swung again. There was an almost immediate upturn in cases and deaths in Vancouver, and many more continued to appear in the surrounding municipalities of Point Grey, South Vancouver, North and West Vancouver, Burnaby, Richmond, and Surrey. No armistice could be signed with the Spanish Lady.

The fight against the flu throughout B.C. had been hampered from the outset by a shortage of medical personnel. The end of the war *did* mean that doctors and nurses would eventually return home, but certainly not in time to have any effect on the battle against the Spanish Lady. That was why volunteers played such an important role in the fight.

Dr. Underhill resisted new pressure from some city fathers and merchants to reopen the city now that the war was over, and he managed to persuade the acting mayor, who had replaced the still-recuperating Gale, to hold off for at least two days in order to determine whether the celebrating crowds on packed city streets had aided and abetted the spread of the disease.

Within days Dr. Underhill had the good news he had waited for: He told reporters there was no sign of a major increase in cases as a result of the November 11 celebrations, but he cautioned that it was premature to reopen the city.

Predictably, Dr. Price chastised Victorians, who not surprisingly had poured out into the streets to celebrate the wonderful victory. He charged that the downtown crowds were responsible for a rise in the incidence of flu, although it was actually impossible to tell if the celebration was to blame. Price's contention that the flu was still a menace and should not be taken lightly was supported by the provincial health department's Dr. Young, who commented, "I do not desire to appear pessimistic but our reports show clearly that the situation is still a serious one and continued care must be taken by the authorities to combat it."

Young's statement was reinforced when the government received a report from W.E. Ditchburn, superintendent of Indian affairs, stating that the epidemic was causing "havoc" among Natives in the interior. A woman named Edith Menzies gave her life trying to help the Native people. She wasn't a trained nurse, but she and her sister, Belle, volunteered to go from the Lower Mainland to Merritt to care for the sick Aboriginal people in the region. Flu killed her a few weeks after she arrived.

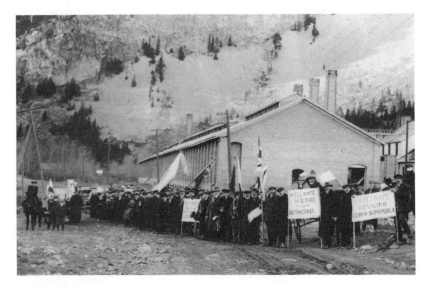

People in communities everywhere, in major cities and in small hamlets, gathered to celebrate the war's end, in spite of dire warnings from public health officials.

There were innumerable acts of kindness and charity. One young man hailed as a hero was 17-year-old Charlie Philip, a timekeeper at a remote spruce-logging camp on Graham Island in British Columbia's Queen Charlotte Islands. The entire crew except for Charlie was felled by flu, and the teenager, with no medical training, worked night and day nursing his colleagues. Finally the disease caught up with him and turned quickly to pneumonia. When the doctor and two nurses who had volunteered to go to the remote location finally arrived, men called out from their sickbeds, "Go to the boy first ... never mind us but you save the boy." Charlie was lucky; he survived.

Perhaps the fact that the Queen Charlottes were without medical assistance for most of the pandemic was one of the reasons that this area's request for liquor for medicinal purposes was successful. Attorney General Farris twice authorized additional cases of brandy and whiskey to be shipped north.

The popularity of spirits increased as the days grew shorter and the Christmas holiday drew nearer. Existing supplies had been expended on November 11. Dr. A.L. Briggs, an American working in Vancouver, was charged and fined $100 for "issuing a prescription for liquor too promiscuously." He obviously was far from alone in his "promiscuousness." Later reports revealed that in the weeks before Christmas, some 700 certificates had been granted to "cheerful invalids."

In mid-November the Association of Theatrical Employees, representing 1,000 entertainers, finally took action to help its members. For four weeks they had been without wages. They had complained individually that they were not being fairly treated, saying that if closure was helping beat the flu, it should be a complete shutdown and not a half-hearted one. They had pointed out that movie halls and theatres were better ventilated than many of the premises that had stayed open. For some time their arguments had fallen on deaf ears.

Frustrated by its members' inability to influence the powers that be, the association did some quiet checking on its own and revealed its findings in a large newspaper advertisement displayed as an open letter to the mayor and the provincial government. It stated that on a recent Saturday afternoon its observers had counted 53 people jammed into a store offering bargain prices on merchandise at a special sale. On the same Saturday night, there were exactly 93 men packed into a city saloon, allegedly drinking only the near-beer permitted by law, "their arms around each other's necks and singing in each other's faces, the glasses were dipped in cold water or more often not washed at all as they passed from mouth to mouth."

The association was by now very short of funds, but it pointed out that its members didn't want charity, they wanted work. The ad pleaded, "Will any doctor come forward and tell us how flu is transmitted or what it is?" Unfortunately, doctors didn't have the answers they wanted. The theatrical workers had public opinion on their side, though. People were tired of wartime austerity and were looking for a chance to laugh and be entertained.

Vancouver reopens

Spurred by the entertainment-industry protest and the apparent abatement of the disease, Vancouver City Council held a special meeting on November 18 that included Underhill and other officials. The meeting approved a motion calling for an end to the closures, and a message was sent to Victoria requesting permission to do so. Provincial Secretary S.D. MacLean immediately assigned Dr. Young to review the situation, and Young caught the midnight boat to Vancouver. He remained leery, but was persuaded by Gale and Underhill that the ban could be lifted. He gave his approval, but warned that new cases would be carefully monitored in case closure must again be imposed. It was November 19, and the bright lights of the city hadn't twinkled for a month.

The papers said there was immediate "joy," even though proprietors also claimed bitterly that the shutdown had cost them $100,000. They were more than ready to reopen, having carefully cleaned up and prepared for the day they had long been anticipating. Lights once again blazed in live theatres and in movie houses, where silver screens flickered. Excited crowds flocked to the Orpheum Theatre, the Vancouver Opera House, Pantages Theatre, and the Empress Theatre to watch the performances of entertainers finally back at work, including Reno, the eccentric tramp cyclist, and Countess de

Leonardi and her troupe, singing excerpts from Pagliacci. A *Sun* critic wrote: "The programs offered were of an unusually effective nature while the various orchestras contributed rousing patriotic selections which found a ready response in every heart." The click of pool and billiard balls could also be heard through the doors of brilliantly lit amusement halls, and from bowling alleys came rumbling sounds as "trundlers" mobilized.

Everyone seemed convinced that the flu was finally on the run. Hordes of people jammed the sidewalks at Granville and Hastings streets, turning out for the one-dollar specials offered on the first Saturday late-night shopping since restricted hours were introduced. Despite the almost overpowering smell of disinfectant, streetcars were packed as they carried happy bargain hunters into town. Caution was thrown to the wind as the housebound population broke loose.

The school board decided that students would not return to class immediately, in order to give teachers who had taken on volunteer nursing duties during the closure another few days to prepare for classes. Chairman W.H. Lang questioned the wisdom of reopening, but most of his colleagues favoured it. Lang stated, "The epidemic is not dead yet and I think you will find a recurrence." He pointed to reports from the U.K. that said a second wave of flu had struck three months after the first attack and was much more severe than the first.

Role of valiant nurses

As the city reopened for business, *The Vancouver Daily Sun* ran the names of 17 sisters and nursing students who had died tending the sick. St. Paul's Sister Superior commented: "I can not say too much of their bravery. They did wonderfully well." The story described them as "Heroines All," women who had given their lives caring for the sick in hospitals and homes. There were many others in Vancouver and throughout the province, but a full list was never compiled, nor was the oft-repeated suggestion that a memorial to them be created ever implemented. The odd plaque was raised—a ward was named for one nurse in a new Nanaimo hospital—but never a significant monument to their memory. Some of the victims were student nurses barely out of their teens. Some travelled far and gave their lives caring for the sick in logging camps, mining communities, and Aboriginal settlements throughout B.C. The Registered Nurses Association of B.C. is among those who would like to have all of those who died listed for the historical record. It continues to add names whenever they are identified.

Reporter Mary Clendenan wrote the story that accompanied the newspaper list. In the style and language of the times, in a long and glowing description, she compared these women to the men who had gone to the front and made the ultimate sacrifice. They were, she wrote, equally brave. Nobody disagreed.

> During the influenza epidemic it was put to
> the women of Vancouver that here was their
> opportunity to serve others at the price of hardship
> and risk to themselves, even as it was put up to the
> men four years ago last August when volunteers
> were called to go to the aid of France and Belgium.
>
> The hardship and risks were less in this case
> but they existed nevertheless, and they had to
> be faced without the moral support of cheering
> comrades and the inspiration of bands and flags.
> The women must come to grips with death in the
> isolated sickroom and must fight the fight alone.
>
> But they accepted the challenge with the
> same splendid promptness that their brothers had
> shown, and the result is that Canada has another
> honour role to which British Columbia alone has
> contributed 17 names, with possibly others not yet
> counted, nurses who died of influenza contracted
> while at their posts of duty. Many of them brought
> their patients to convalescence, but stayed on duty
> too long after getting the infection themselves, and
> so were unable to fight off the disease from which
> they had saved others. Besides the nurses who died
> of the malady, a great many were dangerously ill.
>
> When the epidemic began it was to the
> health authorities, the doctors and the nurses,

that the public looked to, to lead the war upon the disease. In this situation the graduate nurses were somewhat in the position of the few, but expertly trained regulars who formed the nucleus of the vast volunteer army organized to make war upon the Kaiser's hordes. It was taken for granted that they should be the first into the breach, and very heroically they accepted the part. There was heroism on the part of the volunteers also. They were not trained to nurse. Those who were able to volunteer might have sidestepped and made plausible enough excuses. There was many a loophole open to the women who wanted to escape by it. Therefore tribute is being paid at the city hospital and in hundreds of private homes throughout the city to the untrained volunteers who came forward and did what they could.

Between these two classes came the nurses in training at the hospitals and they too have won the name of heroines. They saw so much that they could do to relieve suffering and many begged to remain on duty much longer than their regular hours. A girl who had been in training only a few months actually cried one night because she did not want to leave her patients even to get her needed sleep. About four in the morning she woke in a chill and then her temperature mounted rapidly. Another nurse hurriedly dressed over her night clothes, got medicine and hot water bottles and worked on the girl until it was time to go on duty the next morning. This second nurse never did finish that broken sleep and never did take time all day to undress and dress again in the ordinary manner, her uniform covering a multitude of eccentricities in her costume. This is only one example of service gladly given with never a thought of self.

A third nurse who had been ill was so anxious
to get back to her work that she returned too soon
against the advice of her family and doctor with
the result that her heroism cost her life, for she
suffered a relapse from which she could not rally.

The same spirit prevailed among the graduate
nurses in hospitals and private homes. There are
several instances in which they stayed on duty after
getting the infection, only giving in when on the
point of delirium.

The volunteers played up to the example set
by the regular nurses. Scores of the schoolteachers,
dozens of college girls, and many women without
exacting home ties, did eight-hour duty in the
emergency hospital opened in connection with the
Vancouver General Hospital. Many a business girl
and busy housewife who could not give full time
went into a private home to help for two or three
hours after her regular day's work was done. There
were cases in which a woman dropped her home
duties at a moment's warning and within half an
hour of receiving the call for aid was installed as a
volunteer nurse in some afflicted house.

Clendenan finished her story with quotes from Vancouver
General's Dr. McEachern, Sister Superior Mederic (M. Veronique
Trundel) at St. Paul's, and city relief superintendent Ireland, lauding
those who had given their lives and all who had cared for the citizens
of Vancouver.

There were many stories of the ordeals suffered by all the nurses
and volunteers. Lillian Estabrooks, quoted in the introduction to
this book, was 16 and her sister, Kay, 18, when they responded to a
call to help nurse in a schoolroom-turned-hospital in Hedley in the
B.C. interior. For untrained teenagers, they displayed tremendous
compassion and courage.

Sister Marie Louise St. Jacques was a newly arrived nursing sister
at St. Paul's in 1916; she contracted the flu while caring for the sick and

Heroines All
(By Mary Clendenan)

To the graduate and volunteer nurses in British Columbia has been given an opportunity to vie with the heroism of the military nurses who went overseas to care for the soldiers, in fact the percentage of casualties has been several times greater among these heroic women than among the Red Cross Nurses at the front. That they have grasped the opportunity to the full is shown by the following list of those who gave their lives to free their land of plague.

Sister St. Jacques, died at St. Paul's hospital, Oct. 19.

Sister Syncletique, died at St. Paul's hospital, Oct. 27.

Miss Marjorie Beatrice Moberley, died at Coquitlam Military hospital where she had been nursing influenza patients.

Miss Agnes Atterley Jean Chambers, cared for C.W. Nunley and after his death nursed the sick family until within twenty-four hours of her own death.

Miss C. Patterson, a graduate of Newton, Mass., contracted the disease while nursing influenza patients.

Miss Laura F. Crawford, a graduate of Vancouver General hospital, died at Anyox where she had been nursing.

Miss Ruth B. Luno, a member of the Nelson school staff, volunteered as an assistant at the Vancouver General hospital and also nursed members of her own family.

Miss Edith Menzie, of Pitt Meadows, who had been nursing Indians at Merritt.

Miss Ruth Murphy, who died at Agassiz after she had nursed relatives there to convalescence.

Miss Kathleen Bryant, who had been nursing at St. Paul's hospital but died at her own home.

The remaining six were also nurses in training there:

Miss Marlon Robertson.

Miss Grace Perrin.

Miss Florence Ferrara.

Miss Pearl Williams.

Miss Eulalia Lanoville.

Miss R. Hinde.

Miss Irene Jones.

—from *Vancouver Daily Sun*

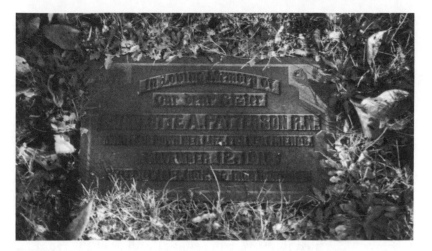

One of the nurses who died during the 1918 flu epidemic was Charlotte Patterson, whose grave is located in Mountain View Cemetery along with those of many others who died of the flu in October and November 1918. Her name is listed as one of those honoured by the city for their service to their patients.

died in 1918. Marjorie Fulmer, a recent graduate nurse in Vancouver, recalled tending the sick in a city emergency centre with camp cots jammed almost side by side. Of working 12-hour shifts, she said, "We were run off our feet just to keep abreast of our patients, all in such critical condition." Nurse Constance Boyle worked in a Vancouver emergency hospital, looking after mostly middle-aged women. She remembered the physical and emotional strain as they tried to care for and comfort patients who were worrying about their families. It was particularly poignant, she said, because most of the patients knew they weren't going to get better.

Mrs. Ethel Thomson and Mrs. Dorothy Pierce D'Arcy-Goldrick were both young nurses during the onslaught. Many years later, they remembered people "dying like flies, unending shifts that lasted from 7 a.m. to 7 p.m. and even longer." Medical staff did what they could with limited options, and the nurses vividly recalled slapping mustard plasters on patients in the hope they would do some good.

Nurse Betty Cox could never forget the searing-hot poultices, a mustard mixture that was spread like peanut butter onto pieces of cotton. "We'd put one on the front and one on the back in bad cases. The idea was by putting heat into the chest, it would bring lots of blood to that area and carry off the disease," she said. It was primitive treatment of questionable value, but these were desperate times. Despite the best care and caution in applying these scalding mixtures, some patients bore traces of burn marks on their skin for the rest of their lives.

With the reopening of Vancouver, more friends and relatives turned out regularly to greet and cheer the returning soldiers. There was a large turnout of friends and family at the railway station late in November to welcome home two of the six brothers of a well-known Vancouver family. All six had fought in the war: One of them, Roderick, had been killed, while majors Alan and Malcolm Bell-Irving had been decorated for bravery in action. Reading of the return of these two heroes was another poignant reminder to the Underhills of the loss of their own two sons in France. Their boys had been acquaintances of the Bell-Irvings in their youth.

Newspapers also reported that the numbers of returning soldiers had produced a housing shortage, which was expected to get much worse before it improved. In an amazing burst of generosity, Ottawa announced that each veteran would be given $65 to buy new clothes.

Victoria reopens

Lifting the closures in Vancouver put so much pressure on Dr. Price that he was forced to accede to the reopening of Victoria. The lights came on again in the capital, and everyone was happy except the medical health officer. He maintained that it was the wrong decision, but it had been imposed on him by the Vancouver move. Price did say that the general flu scene seemed improved. He still advised the public to avoid mingling in crowds, although many ignored his warning.

Joy at the return of the good old days soared with the announcement of an Armistice Ball to be held in Victoria on November 28 in the Empress Hotel, with dancing in the ballroom and the rotunda. Lifting the ban on gatherings had paved the way for some real celebrations. When Professor Louis Turner and his augmented 12-piece orchestra struck up the music, it was in a ballroom decorated with flags of all the

Allied nations, and many gentlemen appeared in their dress uniforms. *The Daily Colonist* reported that John Hart was master of ceremonies and E.N. Hink and Miss Eva Hart led the grand march. A reporter noted, "Almost every innovation and picturesque creation that the ingenious mind could design was represented in the gay, colourful scene." It is not known whether Price decided to waltz the night away or whether he avoided the crowds.

As November ran out, there were ominous signs of a second wave of the disease. Underhill stressed that the flu was still a dire emergency, with the death toll at 562. J.J. Banfield, head of the VGH board, told members that the fatality rate at the hospital and at the emergency units operating at the King Edward was 11 percent. This was much lower than in many other cities, where in some instances it was at a startling 50 percent.

As the number of cases once again began to climb, Mayor Gale said the city would have to reassess the situation and make sure hospitals were geared to receive new patients. He told reporters there was an apparent increase in the number of young children affected and that in one room of 45 students just recently returned to school, 25 were absent due to flu and other ailments. Underhill strongly repeated his opposition to any further shutdown of schools. He also said there would be a renewed search for hotel accommodation for transients who were not sick enough to be hospitalized.

In many other cities, the end of the pandemic was more severe than the beginning, but in Vancouver, the increase in new cases was not as bad; suddenly, for no apparent reason, the situation improved. The change, however, was slow to be felt in hospitals, and one VGH nurse was lucky to escape with her life during a violent flu-related incident. Press reports said she was attacked by F. Tuxen Hartmann, a Norwegian patient delirious with the flu. He stabbed at her with a knife, cutting her uniform but not wounding her. An attendant who rushed to help was hit on the head with a bottle grabbed by the demented man. Hartmann was restrained and put in a straitjacket. Some hours later he was removed from the jacket when he appeared to have calmed, but he then grabbed a razor blade, cut his wrists, and bled to death before anything could be done. The Spanish Lady had claimed another victim.

The Rotary Club gave itself a pat on the back for the volunteer taxi service it had manned to drive doctors, nurses, and visitors to Vancouver hospitals. Their work was much better than the dreadful piece of trivia that made it onto the front page of *The Vancouver Daily Sun* under the headline "Good Work, Rotary." Presumably composed by a Rotarian, it read:

> Say men, this epidemic is wearing off our smiles,
> We have simply got to fight it in true Rotarian style,
> And if you are in a quandary, wondering just what you
>   can do,
> Come and join our 'Fleet of Flying Flivvers Fighting Flu.'
>
> There's Tom and Art and Scott and Lorne and William,
> They've been delivering nurses by the millions,
> While Al and Sanford, Fred and Alex too,
> Are all in our 'Fleet of Flying Flivvers Fighting Flu.'
>
> Ask Jack Watson how the early morning air,
> Puts pep into your day's work and in your heart a prayer,
> He'll tell you how to help us see this blasted thing through,
> By serving in our 'Fleet of Flying Flivvers Fighting Flu.'
>
> We hope its days are numbered and we have it on the run,
> But there's a lot of service yet and we need you every one.
> So don't renege when called upon but shout right out 'me too,'
> For you're in our 'Fleet of Flying Flivvers Fighting Flu.'

The area's health problems were compounded by a statement from New Westminster's medical health officer, Dr. S.C. McEwen, who said that 11 houses in his city were quarantined because of an outbreak of diphtheria. He said the disease seemed to have been contained and there was no need for panic, but warned the public to watch for symptoms, particularly sore throats.

Several newspapers picked up a story contending that the U.S. surgeon general's office had issued a statement claiming they had found the "absolute cure," a mixture of spirits of alcohol and chloroform on a cotton ball that a sufferer could breathe while holding it between the teeth. To most, the suggestion was absolute nonsense, but there is little doubt that a few people tried it.

In late November Dr. J.S.W. McCullough, the chief medical officer for Ontario, released some chilling figures of the terrible death toll in the first six weeks of the epidemic in that province—figures that increased in a later final tally. Based on deaths per 100,000, McCullough's figures showed that Kingston paid the highest price, followed by Toronto, Ottawa, Windsor, and London. Dr. J.A. Beaudry, inspector general for the Quebec Board of Health, also released new figures showing that his province lost 9,925 people, 3,100 of them from Montreal alone.

In Toronto, statistics proved that the Spanish flu had targeted younger men. The tally for the first 167 deaths in the city showed age groups and the fatalities within them: under age 10, 8 deaths; 11 to 20, 18; 21 to 30, 63; 31 to 40, 54; 41 to 50, 20; over 50, 4. A greater number of 20- to 40-year-old men had gone off to war than from any other age bracket; even more men from this age group who stayed home were taken by the Spanish Lady. Later figures from New York confirmed that more than 60 percent of its dead were between 15 and 45 years of age, and that the age of the greatest number of victims was 28.

Flu slowly wanes

By December 8 only five or six new cases a day were being treated at Victoria's Fort Street emergency hospital, considerably fewer than in November, and Dr. Price conceded that the worst was over. A week before Christmas, Price said there had been 2,439 reported cases in Victoria. The actual total was probably higher because many people in the Chinese community did not come forward. Price said 80 nurses and volunteers in Victoria had contracted the flu, and 128 people had volunteered to assist.

The flu's retreat was celebrated in verse—many more people in 1918 spent their leisure time penning poetry than do today. One of these enthusiastic amateurs was Mrs. A. Wilson. Despite its being doggerel, the *Colonist* published a poem of hers entitled "The Spanish Flu":

Oh, the grippe; this terrible grippe,
Thro' country and town it is taking a trip;
Bringing to all a most fearful attack,
Of biliousness, headache and pains in the back.
Its victims are many, its ravages grave;
Its "grippe" is like iron, we lie and we rave,
Groaning and moaning with exquisite pain.
And praying we never may have it again

But one thing I've noticed that this "Spanish Flu"—
Is not a respecter of persons—have you?
It visits the homes of the humble and great
And travels all over the country and state.
Brave men fall before it, proud women as well,
And children have also been smitten and fell.
For one who has come, saw, and conquered all through,
We take off our hats to you, Conquering Flu.

But we don't bid you welcome, Oh, you Mighty Flu.
There's nobody wants you so kindly skidoo.
At your word of command we have closed every door,
Of theatres, movies, and places galore.
You've shut down our meetings and even our schools,
You've treated us just like a parcel of fools.
And even our churches and Sunday schools too,
You've closed with a bang, Oh, you wonderful Flu!

Still, altho' you have made us obey every whim,
We rise up in defiance, your chance is now slim.
We'll chase you before us, grim spectre away!
We'll fear you no longer, we'll route you today.
You've stalked through our midst like a fiend seeking prey,
'Til you quite overpowered our brightest and gay,
But your day is near over, you've had us, 'tis true,
And we are the conquerors, Oh, Great Spanish Flu.

With Christmas festivities underway and a growing feeling among the public that the crisis was over, Underhill warned against complacency—31 new deaths were recorded for December. "It is inviting trouble when the public does not take ordinary sanitary precautions," he stated. He was annoyed that spitting in public was again becoming common, and he also had the usual bee in his bonnet about dancing and cautioned residents to steer clear of all large events, private and public. He contended that dancing overheated the body, and then revellers exposed themselves to drafts when they sat near open windows during the streetcar trip home. His other warnings for the Christmas season included: Try to avoid crowds in stores, guard against wearing wet clothing; keep the feet dry.

Entertainment-starved residents, however, continued to crowd cinemas to see all their favourites, from Charlie Chaplin and Douglas Fairbanks to Theda Bara and Billie Burke, along with all the ever-popular cowboy stars.

The first post-war Christmas was a time of rejoicing and, for those who had lost loved ones, of sadness. Christmas carols rang through well-attended churches, and carollers carried their songs into the streets, where many houses were gaily decorated with lights and greenery. Amidst the festivities, many people were caring for the broken veterans who had made it back from the front, wounded in body or spirit, sometimes both. Flu still took no holiday and often struck these brave survivors.

Private Herbert Bradley had concealed his age and enlisted in the army at the age of 15. He was gassed and wounded fighting at Vimy Ridge; on his way home, he caught the flu and was carried off by the Spanish Lady. He was a son of Sergeant-Major Harold Bradley, who was still overseas. Private Bradley had two brothers in France, and a third brother had been sent home suffering from shellshock.

There was no longer the same shortage of beds as there had been during the early weeks of the pandemic. A new emergency hospital at VGH was completed early in the new year, providing space for 150 beds. However, the Spanish Lady had not yet departed. VGH lost two more staff members. Dr. Daniel Mahoney was only 34. He was the hospital's assistant superintendent and had been working round the clock since the beginning of the epidemic. He was a graduate of Queen's University in Kingston, Ontario, and had been in B.C.

for only 18 months. Superintendent McEachern lauded Mahoney's work, saying the young doctor's performance during the epidemic had been of unequalled excellence. A younger victim, Grace Hopkins, was one of the hospital's student nurses; she had been in training for two years and died tending the sick. Grace was from a well-known B.C. family, which gave its name to Hopkins Landing, a picturesque community on Howe Sound.

As 1918 ended, authorities began to look at the unprecedented death toll. Vancouver officials said the pandemic accounted for a large part of the 2,405 people who had died during the year. The total for the previous year was 1,549.

The early breakdown of deaths by region showed: Vancouver, 778; Victoria, 127; Nanaimo, 143; Alberni, 188; Ashcroft, 69; Fairview (covering the Prince George area), 175; and Beaton (the Kootenays), 340. Vancouver's total was much higher than the other regions because of the large population in the Lower Mainland and because of the large number of patients who had come there seeking treatment.

If the overall death toll in Canada was bad, it was staggering in other parts of the world. In the last 12 weeks of 1918 alone, more than six million people died worldwide, and many more than that had died earlier in the year. There were more than 32,000 fatalities in England and Wales. Undertakers in London were unable to take care of the huge number of bodies needing burial, and coffins were stacked waiting to be placed in the ground. London officials said that more than three million people had died in recent months in India, and this figure could be low by as much as several million because of poor statistical reporting in that country. At the peak of the pandemic, nearly 800 died daily in Delhi, a city that at the time had a population of 200,000 people.

In the new year, Dr. Young warned B.C. Premier John Oliver that the flu was still a "serious problem." As a result, a special meeting was called for provincial and municipal health representatives from around the province. Dr. Underhill spoke for many of the health officers in attendance when he said that if the disease recurred there should be a total shutdown of stores, offices, and all the factories that had been permitted to remain open originally. Vancouver had been the only B.C. city with a significant number of factories operating during the fall of 1918. Doctors in all districts now agreed that the partial closure had been ineffective. Underhill's contention that a partial closure was useless had been vindicated.

The medical men also agreed that in the event of the flu's return, there should be a bigger and more co-ordinated public information campaign to tell all residents exactly what was happening and what preventive measures they should take—the very step that Underhill had unsuccessfully pressed for prior to the Spanish Lady's arrival in Vancouver.

Underhill's lifelong advocacy of handwashing as a prime factor in the fight against the spread of infectious diseases was also fully endorsed at the meeting, and the veteran doctor was strongly supported in his insistence that the no-spitting rule be enforced. Nobody was laughing now at these mundane measures; they were stressed again for the public.

Always a man to stay well ahead of the crowd, Underhill used every opportunity to expound on his views and try to improve areas

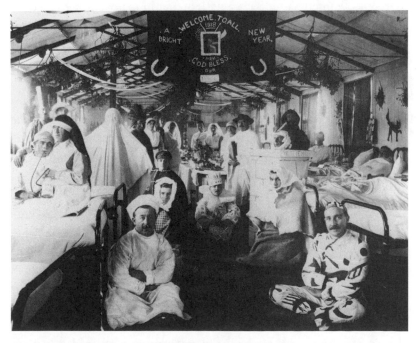

Wounded veterans had something to celebrate for New Year's 1918: They had not died from influenza. Pictured here is a New Year's party in a war hospital in France.

of the city where he felt there were health issues. He emphasized to reporters that there was an urgent need to clean up Vancouver, which he said had become filthy while everyone's efforts were concentrated on tackling the flu. He also kicked off a new campaign that he hoped to introduce in the city's restaurants. He wanted owners to sterilize their equipment, because it would reduce the number of customers who became ill from eating contaminated food.

British Columbians were confronted, in the coldest days of winter, with reports of the anticipated second wave of the flu. All the signs were there, as the death count rose again. Only weeks into the New Year another 37 died in Vancouver. Doctors across Canada and abroad insisted that this wave of pandemic flu was different from the first strain; it was characterized by a more severe final-stage pneumonia, which developed into a sort of "blood poisoning" that was fast, fatal, and almost impossible to counteract. A large number of victims developed a throat swelling that quickly poisoned the entire body. Sometimes early and vigorous treatment could save a patient, but in many cases it failed.

Suddenly, the renewed closure discussed by the provincial committee was close to becoming a reality. As always, there were those who disagreed, and this time a delegation of churchmen rushed to the capital to urge exemption for places of worship.

While this second wave of flu proved less lengthy and less contagious, it was, nonetheless, claiming too many victims. The ambulance service in Vancouver put more vehicles into service, and the indefatigable Underhill continued his cleanliness crusade, convinced that any flu was a case of "hand-to-mouth" transmission.

Once again disinfectant supplies dwindled and prices soared. Gouging was criticized as the cost of camphor went from 40 cents a pound to $6.50. At a council meeting, alderman Frank Woodside underlined the problem of the "high cost of dying." He had received a letter from an irate constituent who complained that undertakers were making a good thing out of a bad situation, charging $100 for caskets that should have sold for $35.

In the end, city council did not order a new closure, but towards the end of January the provincial government ordered a ban on all private and public dances, believing that while some halls had proper ventilation, others did not. The decision must have pleased

Underhill, if indeed he hadn't pushed Victoria into such action. As anticipated, there were complaints from all directions.

Mayor Gale hurried to say it was the province, not the city, that had imposed the ban "on dance halls and terpsichorean entertainment." Alderman Hoskins said during the debate that he wasn't a dancer, but "I like to see them swinging in the corners." Musicians, once again out of work, complained that the move was totally unnecessary since the pandemic obviously was on the wane. They also claimed that most of the public believed the same thing. Everyone was relieved when the ban didn't last long.

McEachern told the VGH board that 13,375 patients had been treated in 1918, at an average cost of $2.31 each, a three-cent increase over the previous year. There were also 352 flu fatalities, and a deficit of $21,123, much of it attributable to the pandemic.

With teachers and medical workers the most affected by the siege of the Spanish Lady, it wasn't long before negotiations began to increase the wages of both. In addition, the Vancouver Teachers' Association asked for an annual $1,000 minimum wage. Salaries at this time were $780 for a new schoolteacher and $1,140 for a teacher with seven years' experience. Male high school teachers would now get $1,560 after the first year and $2,400 after eight years. With blatant discrepancy an acceptable part of the system, female teachers doing the same job got about $200 less. A school nurse in her first year was paid $840 annually.

In his annual report, Teachers' Board chairman W.H. Lang paid tribute to the school doctors, nurses, teachers, and other staff who had volunteered to help fight the flu, "some of whom gave their lives in this noble work."

In February, the fact that the flu was a worldwide sickness was underlined by its arrival in far-off Australia, isolated by distance because sea voyages from Europe or North America to Down Under took many weeks. The flu's appearance triggered a violent internal debate. The state of Victoria bore the brunt of the attack, the international press reporting some 600 cases and 30 deaths, while the flu wasn't as bad in neighbouring New South Wales. This led to bitter disputes when inspectors appeared at state borders to check travellers. Tempers flared and these actions were criticized as a "most serious issue"—all of this taking place little more than 15 years after Australia's separate states had agreed to become one country.

There was a call for a worldwide conference on the "baffling flu" in London, where authorities said most major cities in the U.K. had more than 2,000 dead, with the incidence of disease now highest in Scotland.

Vancouverites continued to meet the trains, often now welcoming wide-eyed war brides as well as returning veterans. On one train was a shipment of Flanders Fields poppies brought to the city and planted in Stanley Park. The true cost of war was reflected when Private T.W. Collins returned to Powell River, the only one alive of eight colleagues who had enlisted in 1915.

There was another slight upswing in the incidents of flu early in March, but Dr. McEachern seemed unperturbed, stating that the new emergency building at VGH would be closed and turned over to the military at the end of the month if cases continued to decline. By April the flu was definitely on the wane; the disease was still active, but fewer people were dying.

In his report for the year McEachern stated that VGH had treated 14,047 patients, of whom 887 had died. The number of patients had peaked on October 25, when the hospital accommodated 1,304 sick people. The Infants' Hospital at 1154 Bute Street reported that there were four cases of influenza in babies under two and 16 cases of pneumonia. The superintendent paid a tribute to his staff, stating, "I feel I cannot express in appropriate words my deepest appreciation of the excellent contribution of the entire staff during the year and especially through the disastrous epidemic of influenza which we have passed."

Life began to return to normal. May was quiet, and by June the Spanish Lady appeared to have left town. Vancouver, under the vigilant eye of Dr. Underhill, had paid a heavy price for the Lady's visit, but the toll was much less than in other parts of Canada and around the world. The battle apparently over, the tireless health officer resumed his campaign to ensure pure water, clean streets, hygienic food stores and restaurants, and to continue the search for procedures to improve the overall health of his community.

DEVASTATION FAR AND WIDE

Vancouver, the Lower Mainland, and Victoria suffered the largest number of cases and fatalities during the time when the flu seemed to be everywhere, but few corners of the province escaped the Spanish Lady's clutches. Towns large enough to have hospitals had trained doctors and nurses to help them, but smaller locations had to cope as best they could, each settlement or family on its own. In the case of remote villages, help was slow to arrive, and often it never came at all. It is doubtful whether all of those who suffered and died were ever identified or included in the overall tally of losses. The tally was not a priority for those trying to save still-living friends and family.

The Spanish Lady had arrived initially in Corbin, a small, lusty, coal-mining town near the Crowsnest Pass in the Kootenay Mountains. As the crow flies, it is about mid-way between Fernie, B.C., and Pincher Creek, Alberta. In 1918, Corbin's immigrant population was sustained by the heavy demands of the railways in Canada and the U.S. for the coal found in the shiny black seams of rock that stretched deep into the craggy cliffs surrounding the town. There was work for anyone who wanted it in 1918, the money was good in the mines, and there was the option of making bootleg booze at one of the stills tucked carefully away in the mountains. Everyone worked hard and played hard in Corbin.

This lifestyle was abruptly interrupted at the beginning of October when the trains that had made the town rich brought in unwanted baggage. Within days the Spanish flu afflicted the heart of the community and curtailed mining production. Even the stills shut down when half of the community's population took to their beds.

Corbin's medical facilities were meagre, and the only doctor was one of the first to be taken ill. His advice to townsfolk before becoming too sick to care for them was to "stay in bed, take Epsom salts and more Epsom salts." With the doctor out of commission, the mine manager took the situation in hand and, assisted by some of his foremen, made the rounds to check on employees and neighbours. The mine committee had coal and foodstuffs delivered to those unable to look after themselves, and those people still on their feet volunteered to help the very ill and to make meals.

The town's dance hall was converted into an emergency hospital for sick bachelors. Instead of digging for coal, some of the miners were soon digging graves, as the Spanish Lady claimed her first B.C. interior victims. Pleas were sent to other Kootenay communities for help, but the flu spread so rapidly, there was no one available in this or any other region of the province.

Into the Kootenays

As Corbin struggled with the frightful effects of the flu, the Spanish Lady travelled ever westward through the Rocky and the Columbia mountain ranges, with devastating results. She leapfrogged along the rail line, finding new victims in the towns of Rossland, Fernie, and Trail. Within only a few days 800 cases had been tallied in Fernie, about one person in five forced to take to bed, and the death toll climbed to 60. In Rossland a staggering 500 cases were confirmed, and among the first 50 who died was 34-year-old police chief James McLean. He left a wife and two small children.

The few doctors and nurses in the district worked night and day in what at times seemed a losing battle. Like others before them across the country, they looked for a reason for the terrible losses being suffered in their small, close-knit communities. Some people wondered if the altitude made the disease worse than it was elsewhere, but then they realized that other communities perched even higher on the peaks got off lightly by comparison.

In Trail, one emergency isolation hospital filled quickly, so city council opened another in the old Aldredge Hotel. It, too, was soon packed with patients. This was the heart of B.C.'s mining country, and at one point the workforce was reduced by more than 1,000 miners. Coal production fell drastically, so much so that authorities began to worry if there would be enough coal to meet the heavy winter demands in western Canada, which were met in considerable measure by the Kootenay fields.

Nelson was the centre of the region, and the largest and best equipped to handle the medical emergency. In addition to an old hospital, which was immediately turned into an isolation unit, there was the brand new Kootenay Lake General Hospital, which had opened a week or two earlier in September 1918. Medical Health Officer Dr. Isobel Arthur, one of the first women in the province to hold such a position, commented to a local reporter in the *Nelson Daily News*, "If the people realized the gravity of the situation, they would be only too glad to take all suggested protective measures."

Despite its excellent facilities, the town was hard pressed to deal with the more than 500 cases that developed, and nine people had died by November 9. As an added precaution, Dr. Arthur ordered a two-week-long quarantine at home for all discharged patients. It is not known whether or not the quarantine was successful, but it did not save the town's very new and very popular mayor. R.H. (Mungo) McQuarrie was a 52-year-old businessman whose death resulted in an outpouring of respect and acclaim. He had served his community as mayor for less than one year.

Miss Sadie McCallum was the proud newly appointed matron of Kootenay Lake Hospital, but she was to be another tragic victim, in a family terribly struck by the pandemic. A graduate of St. Paul's Hospital nursing school in Vancouver, she had served in Great Britain until 1916, when she returned to B.C. She had recently taken the newly created position in the Kootenays. She caught the flu and died within days. She was the third member of her family to be stricken; all of them died. Her brother, Sergeant Neil McCallum, 21, died of the flu in France, and her sister, Mrs. Percy Booth of Courtenay, had died only days earlier, leaving behind three children, one of them only two weeks old.

Another Nelson nurse who died was 22-year-old Martha Gertrude Knott. She was an attractive, diminutive young woman who had worked an 18-hour shift and then lain down to rest for a couple of hours. When she awoke, she had developed a cough and fever. She wanted to return to her duties, but was told to stay in bed. She replied, "I am alright, I am strong. I must look after my patients." It was not to be.

By mid-November, the hospital was having difficulty coping because so many nurses were sick, and the *Nelson Daily News* implored volunteers to help at the hospital, proclaiming in a headline: "The need is very great, volunteer at once."

Cranbrook's hospital had been built in 1900, and the town was proud of its Tudor architectural style and the facilities it provided, but it was soon overwhelmed with flu cases. An old hotel, The Wentworth, had to be reopened as an emergency facility. Nurses ministered to residents, including the staff of the local paper, *The Cranbrook Herald.* When the linotype operator was stricken, the few remaining employees set type by hand to keep readers informed of the progress of the epidemic.

A few smaller communities escaped the flu altogether; Sandon kept its number of cases to one. It was one of five mining towns in the "silvery Slocan," located midway between Kaslo and New Denver. City fathers held a meeting in the opera house when they learned the flu was getting close and refused to let anyone get off the train when it passed through. The one suspected victim was isolated immediately and may actually have had only a bad cold. Now a ghost town and tourist attraction with a population of six, Sandon had about 5,000 inhabitants at the time of the epidemic.

Kamloops and Kelowna

There was one interior B.C. city well prepared for the onslaught of the Spanish Lady. Early in the fall, Dr. J.T. Robinson, chairman of the Royal Inland Hospital Board in Kamloops, had personally experienced the devastation the Lady could cause when he travelled with his family to Toronto. The city was in turmoil, all its hospitals were overcrowded, and hundreds were dying when Robinson's wife and two daughters fell ill. Unable to find hospital beds for them, he nursed them back to health in their rooms at the King Edward Hotel.

Following their recovery, he hurried back to B.C. and called an urgent meeting of the hospital board. Robinson warned that the pandemic was on the move and would soon reach Kamloops. When it arrived he wanted the town to be well prepared, and it was. The hospital ward was stocked and made ready to handle a large influx of patients. Extra cots were secured and set up wherever they could be fitted in. A vacant building on Nicola Street became a secondary facility. Finally, knowing the number of beds available was still inadequate, the board obtained the use of the Patricia Hotel on Victoria Street, converted it into a hospital, and had it completely staffed by the time the epidemic reached its peak in the community. A separate facility was also set up at the army barracks to accommodate the Aboriginal people, who wanted to minister to their own as much as possible.

Fortunately, Robinson himself never did contract the flu— probably he had become immune to it while he was in Toronto. Throughout the epidemic he was likened to a full-time general, totally in charge of the situation. Other board members did not fare so well. W.T. Summers, of Summers and Frost Clothing Store, chairman of the house committee, was desperately afraid of catching the flu but did not let his fear affect his volunteer activities and stayed on duty until he could no longer stand on his feet. To the dismay of his friends, he died within days of taking to his bed.

James P. Gillespie, manager of the Imperial Bank, and William Brennan were the board members in charge of providing transportation and procuring nurses. The hospital was soon at its 80-patient capacity, with children accommodated in cots in the hall. By the time the patient count climbed to 245, it was a night-and-day job to find cooks, engineers, and the other personnel needed to keep the place functioning. Once the Patricia Hotel was ready, the two men spent much of their time touring the district, urging any who could be spared to help out. At one point, as the disease raged on, the Patricia Hospital lost three matrons in five days. Nurses worked until they were so tired they could scarcely stand, and some became too weak to fight off the disease. Many were out of action for up to 10 days, their experience lost in the struggle.

Dr. H.L. Burris of the Burris Clinic in Kamloops explained: "The doctors were never at rest. When one had a call to the country, he would sleep both going and coming, in the back seat of his car, with a chauffeur at the wheel. He had a list of calls to be made both in the country and town, and the chauffeur took charge of delivering him to the right home." Doctors' offices were left with a nurse in charge who kept lists of calls to be made and passed on advice relayed from doctors.

From Kamloops the shadow of the Spanish Lady spread south almost overnight, into the Okanagan Valley. The first reported case was in Vernon, and while none were yet confirmed in Kelowna, one family there had already lost a son to the flu. He was Neil McMillan, who had been serving with the army engineers in Niagara Falls. His parents had lost two other sons in the fighting in France. Neil's casket was shipped home, and by the time it arrived there was a local ban on public meetings, including church services. The casket was placed on the lawn beside the family home, where a service was held. Local veterans in uniform carried the casket to the hearse for the ride to the cemetery.

Kelowna doctors had identified 15 possible cases when an isolation hospital was set up in an unused school. One local doctor checking on the small Chinese community in Kelowna found several flu cases and four dead. The people there apparently had been afraid to report the deaths for fear of being accused of bringing the disease into town. All houses involved were quarantined, and in a statement in the *Kelowna Courier,* Chief Constable Thomas announced that Chinese people from out of town would be banned from entering the community. He stated, "The only Chinamen who will be allowed on the streets will be wearing white linen tags bearing a permit."

The old Lum Lock house on Ellis Street was set up as a hospital for the Chinese. They were very superstitious and believed the flu was spread by an evil spirit that had taken the form of a small white boy about six years of age, wearing no shoes or socks. They believed anyone who saw the boy would get the flu, and so they remained indoors in their own homes as much as possible.

The *Kelowna Courier* advised readers to use camphor and quinine in efforts to beat the flu. By November 12, the paper had stated that the outbreak was a thing of the past, and schools shut since mid-October would reopen in a few days. At this time there were only four new cases in the emergency hospital, the Chinese hospital was closed, and a separate Japanese hospital had only four patients.

Kelowna and Penticton escaped the heavy losses suffered in the Kootenays. By October 31 Penticton had only five cases, described as mild, although Medical Health Officer Dr. R.B. White acknowledged that there were several patients from other nearby communities, particularly Summerland and Naramata, who were being treated in hospital in Penticton. The caseload rose to 250, with two deaths. Dr. White had opened an emergency hospital, which he declared was functioning well, and he had received a good volunteer response. Most of the Okanagan escaped the second wave of the flu in December.

In the Cariboo country, accounts reaching Victoria told of a heavy death toll on the Chilcotin and Stoney Creek reserves. Within days the Stoney Creek band was decimated. A Catholic priest, Father Cuccolo, went to minister to them and was appalled at the number who died. Death also struck the Aboriginal people in Lillooet with a savagery not seen since they had become victims of the smallpox brought in by early settlers 50 years earlier. Figures were sketchy and unreliable, but it was estimated that at least eight people a day were dying.

One elderly couple at White Lake in the B.C. interior locked themselves in their small home and wouldn't let anyone in to visit unless the guest was willing to swallow their "warding-off" mixture made of strong tea laced with mustard. Neighbours who periodically checked on the couple were forced to gulp it down in order to gain entry to the house. They commented afterward that it tasted much worse than Ottawa's recommended "eggie drink," a concoction made of a pint of water, the whipped whites of two eggs, salt, and cinnamon.

Suffering in the north

Simultaneously with the Okanagan and Cariboo regions, B.C.'s northern centre in Prince George began its fight against the Spanish Lady. The only town in the region with a hospital, its facilities were almost immediately stretched to the limit. Patients began to arrive from villages in the surrounding area, all seeking the help of the

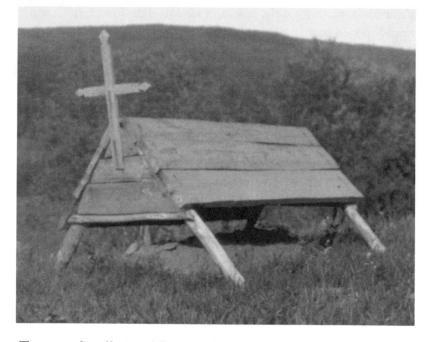

The grave of an Aboriginal flu victim; the influenza virus was particularly devastating for some of the country's First Nations.

only doctors and nurses available to them. By mid-October cases were being sent to the Connaught Hotel, which had been set up as an emergency isolation hospital. The town was closed down almost immediately as the first 22 cases were confirmed, and within four days there were 69.

The RCMP took on the job of trying to find missing trappers and checking on anyone living alone or in an isolated location. One officer commented that there were likely draft dodgers from the war hiding in the area, and he feared some of them might be sick or dead and no one would know. RCMP constables began to arrive with patients from isolated mining camps miles to the north and from Aboriginal families; the latter seemed to suffer much more acutely than others.

The Native population in the northern part of the province, as in the Cariboo, was very badly affected by the flu, and on November 1 the band chief in Fort George died in the first few days of the epidemic. Sub-Chief Joseph Qua was so afraid of the disease that he left the village with his son and daughter to live alone until the danger had passed. He struck a camp several miles up the Fraser River. Some time later, a passerby found all three of them dead in their tent.

In Stewart Lake, 70 Aboriginal people were dead and another 25 were not expected to survive. The *Prince George Citizen* reported, "The epidemic is still raging and apparently has no mercy for the poor Indian." The Pacific Great Eastern Railway helped by shipping food to homes and settlements, many of them Native encampments, along its route. The total death toll among First Nations is difficult to confirm. The South West Indian Inspectorate, representing 21,567 Natives, reported 714 dead, but the numbers were incomplete, as word had not yet been received from 3,500. Another district agent reported 154 dead from a total of 1,400 in his area.

The *Prince George Citizen* lauded the town's two doctors, Drs. Lyon and Lazier, who had treated hundreds of men, women, and children from the region. When Dr. Lyon became too ill to continue, Lazier and his nursing staff laboured on, doing as much as they were able. Locally born Chew Wing was the first Chinese man to die in Prince George.

B.C.'s coast, with its ship traffic, was the only area to feel the brunt of the pandemic as badly as eastern B.C. during the first days of October. In fact, the community of Prince Rupert learned the flu was on the way when they read the *Prince Rupert News* on September 25. The constant arrival of ships from the U.S. brought the illness to B.C.'s major northern port early. In 1918, ships and trains were the major means of transportation, and passenger-ship traffic between San Francisco, Portland, Seattle, Victoria, Vancouver, Prince Rupert, and Alaskan ports was brisk. It was served largely by two major companies, Canadian Pacific's B.C. Coastal Service and the Grand Trunk Pacific, as well as by several smaller lines that helped to handle heavy traffic between June and October. In 1918 their traffic included the Spanish Lady.

Short of beds, nurses, and general help, the St. John Ambulance Association in Prince Rupert went on the hunt for volunteers. The immigration department found 25 unused beds, and these were immediately put to use in the Borden Street School, which was turned into an isolation hospital. It was instantly filled, and Prince Rupert

City Council asked Victoria for help. The city desperately needed five trained nurses and three orderlies, but the minister of health could find no one to send. In a quandary similar to Prince George's, the port city found itself flooded with patients from the hinterland and nearby smaller communities. Every day, fishermen, some near death, tied up at Prince Rupert's docks. One boat contained a whole family—mother, father, and nine children. Eight children survived, left behind as orphans.

Nearby Port Simpson was initially spared from the flu, and the medical missionary there, Dr. P.R. Large, offered his services to Prince Rupert, where he felt he could be of more use. He was welcomed and attended to patients in the regular hospital, as well as in the isolation unit on Borden Street. When the school facility was finally closed late in the year, the *News* lauded "the careful and efficient nursing which had saved several apparently hopeless cases."

Two prominent deaths in Prince Rupert included businessman and alderman R.J.D. Smith and Gus Wick, the popular operator of the local White Lunch restaurant. In another part of town, five Sikh friends worked in the pouring rain to cut five-foot lengths of yellow cedar for the funeral pyre of their fellow lumber worker, Harry Singh, who had died at the emergency hospital. They used coal oil to keep the fire alight in the steady downpour, a lonely group saying farewell to a friend on what seemed a very foreign shore.

Ships of the Consolidated Whaling Company did not return to Prince Rupert until mid-November, avoiding the worst of the pandemic. The fleet reported a catch in 1918 of just one short of 1,000 whales, but fishing that year was generally poor, as many fishermen were ill at the height of the season.

The coastal mining and smelting town of Anyox, 80 miles north of Prince Rupert near the Alaskan border, was a booming centre of activity in 1918, and the constant ship traffic brought the disease to this otherwise isolated community before it reached some interior towns. By October 23 the local doctor had reported 400 cases and 11 deaths. By November 1, the death toll had risen to 44, with 25 dying the preceding day.

News from smaller villages filtered out slowly. At Kitwanga, the Aboriginal "town of totems" on the Skeena River, 16 died during

November. Five people were reported dead in New Hazelton, one in Smithers, and five in Telkwa, "not including Indians."

On Vancouver Island

One of the more astute medical heath officers, Dr. W.F. Drysdale, warned residents of Nanaimo on Vancouver Island early in October that flu was sweeping North America and was bound to arrive in their community soon. The precautions and treatment provided were better than in many other locations, but nonetheless Nanaimo was one of the most severely hit communities. Drysdale's prediction started to come true on October 16 when the first 20 cases were reported.

Drysdale supported the preventive measures recommended by Young and Underhill, and Nanaimo City Council decided to close schools and other public gathering places sooner rather than later. Despite the precautions, within two days there were 135 cases of the flu and the first death: Mrs. Philip Frenchie, a Snuneymuxw woman from the local reserve. As the number of victims climbed and the situation became more critical, council decided to convert the athletic club on Church Street into an emergency hospital. But Nanaimo was treating the area from Ladysmith to Parksville, and even the extra facilities were soon so overcrowded that the home for hospital nurses was set up as a second extra emergency ward. One doctor was also very ill. In only two days the number of cases jumped to 400, with seven deaths and three more doctors ill.

The *Nanaimo Free Press* said that some neighbours were afraid to visit homes where people were sick and suffering, and the hospital board made an appeal for local ladies to make sheets for the emergency hospital. It also requested volunteers for the hospital kitchen. "All that's needed is intelligent and capable hands," the report stressed, but "we must fight the flu with the same determination as the army in France." Doctors now recommended that the sick be treated at home whenever possible because there were no beds left in any of the hospitals.

With many stores and government facilities closed, another outlet was needed to provide liquor for treating Nanaimo's flu patients at home. One doctor said that if liquor was being given to patients in hospital, it should also be of help to patients at home. The provincial government quickly agreed that the local government agent could act as a supplier of alcohol for the duration of the epidemic, providing customers did not gather in groups to obtain it. The rule imposed was one customer at a time.

By November 5 obituaries began to appear in a special column on the front page of the *Free Press*. Council announced a ban on public funerals and urged that people be buried "as quietly as possible." Dr. Drysdale recommended that all funerals be private and small, that no open caskets be allowed, and that burial take place within 72 hours of death.

Gradually the number of cases in Nanaimo began to decline, and although by month's end the death toll had reached 60, the emergency hospital was soon closed. The newspaper said the cost of fighting the epidemic was $10,000. By Christmas Dr. Drysdale announced that the flu emergency was over; it was a welcome gift for a community now permitted to attend religious services, to celebrate the season and to give thanks in the church of their choice.

Late in November, the trans-Pacific cable service was delayed when many of the staff at the Bamfield relay station, on the west side of Vancouver Island, became ill. About the same time, the entire staff at the tiny Campbell River hospital was down with the flu and volunteers were struggling to maintain service.

Early on in the epidemic, Cumberland, which had a large Chinese population, had about 61 cases and one death. Homes in which the illness had struck were placarded. The school, built for the children of early Chinese miners, was turned into a temporary hospital with 20 beds. It was staffed with volunteers organized by the wives of the Anglican minister and the local bank manager. Victoria accommodated a request from the Chinese community for a Chinese doctor, who set up an emergency hospital for the Asian population of Cumberland in the Masonic hall. The doctor found 18 cases and three dead in adjacent Union Bay, where many of the Chinese coal miners now lived. The epidemic resulted in a 25 percent reduction in coal production.

Also on the Island, in the nearby community of Comox, the local newspaper stoutly maintained that despite "pernicious rumours" there was no flu in town. It was a story many found difficult to believe, because by November 21 two men had died of the flu.

In the south

On the south coast, a report from Powell River said more than 200 people had contracted the flu and the forest products mills had been forced to close. Smaller isolated communities and family settlements along B.C.'s rugged coast, previously served only by the vessels of the Columbia Coast Mission, coped as best they could, aided now by a provincial government motor launch that often battled storms to bring medical help and supplies.

Reported about the same time the Fraser Valley town of Chilliwack, like the coastal communities, felt the effects of the flu early. An IODE convention scheduled for October 10 was cancelled. A local merchant, druggist and stationer H.G. Barber, advertised a special treatment for the flu called "the protector." The small bag, which cost 25 cents, contained antiseptics and was to be worn around the neck. Barber also urged customers to buy lots of reading material for their anticipated stays in bed. Chilliwack's medical health officer, Dr. J.C. Henderson, reminded residents that they must report all flu cases and cited heavy penalties if they did not. There were 100 students and five staff sick at the Sardis residential school in Coqualeetza, he said, and the school was being turned into an emergency hospital. There were 20 flu cases in the Asian population of the Dewdney area.

Alaska and Labrador

The two areas of North America that suffered most from the Spanish Lady were rugged, desolate, sparsely populated regions a continent apart: Alaska and Labrador, on the Pacific and Atlantic coasts. The number of deaths amongst the Aboriginal populations in these regions was catastrophic and incomparable to anything experienced anywhere else in North America.

The pandemic arrived in Alaska aboard the passenger ships that plied the Pacific Coast bringing travellers north from San Francisco, Portland, Seattle, Victoria, and Vancouver. In 1918, nearly all goods, services, and people entering or leaving Alaska and Canada's Yukon Territory arrived by sea. From the main entry point of Skagway, the only train travel was on the White Pass and Yukon railway, which ran to Whitehorse. From there travel was by sled or stagecoach.

The population of Alaska at this time comprised 32,000 whites and 23,000 Native Alaskans. In the Yukon, the total population was about 6,000. The number of residents had been declining since the start of the war because so many young men had enlisted and gone overseas. The war and the exodus of people created a severe economic downturn for the whole of the north: Mines had closed and transportation routes were minimized. The Canadian government reduced the number of councillors in the Yukon from 10 to 3; the number of civil servants was reduced correspondingly. There was a severe shortage of trained personnel, particularly doctors. One physician at Nulaka on the Yukon River was the only doctor for 500 miles.

The weather closed in and the annual freeze-up began by mid-October in 1918, shutting down the river routes to interior regions. Anyone who was heading south for the winter was in Skagway by mid- to late October, and there were few if any travellers inbound. This may account for the fact that the Yukon was more fortunate than other areas; while few records are available, the number of flu victims seems to have been lower there than in Alaska.

On October 12 Alaska Governor Thomas Riggs Jr. learned that 75 people in Seattle had died of the flu and the pandemic was spreading fast all along the coast. He ordered steamship companies to refuse passage to anyone who appeared to have symptoms of the flu, for they would not be allowed to land in Alaska. He also assigned a physician to meet each ship to check for sickness. By the end of the month there were 350 dead in Seattle, and Governor Riggs told health officials throughout his territory to refuse entry to anyone from outside who had even the slightest suspicion of sickness.

Despite the governor's precautions, the flu did arrive in Alaska and was particularly severe throughout all the communities in the Panhandle. The first case in Juneau was identified on October 14, and by the end of the month the disease was spreading rapidly, unstopped by the closure of schools and theatres and the cancellation of all public meetings.

One of the most affected centres in Alaska was the isolated community of Nome, and yet the precautions taken to prevent the spread of the epidemic there were particularly stringent. The ship *Victoria* left Seattle in mid-October; three doctors had examined the passengers to ensure that no one was ill. She arrived in Nome on October 20, still with no sickness aboard. All passengers were then quarantined for five days, and all mail and freight was fumigated. The *Victoria* was the last ship of the season and was the only vessel to dock at Nome that month, yet on the return voyage 153 passengers became ill; 47 were rushed to hospital on arrival in Seattle, and 30 of them died by the end of November.

Just like the ship, Nome could not escape the flu; the devastation was almost unbelievable. The disease spread like wildfire and within days moved on into the Native villages on the outskirts of the community. The *Victoria* was the last contact with the outside world for the whole of the Seward Peninsula that fall season. She brought the Spanish Lady and left communities there with no hope of aid from the outside. Inhabitants faced months of sickness and death in the total isolation and darkness of an arctic winter. The pandemic raged unchecked. Few Natives in the area escaped; 162 died during a one-week period. They seemed to be extremely vulnerable: 700 in a very small population on the peninsula died.

The maritime quarantine did save a few small communities in Alaska, but by November the Spanish Lady was much in evidence in centres from Nome to St. Michael on the Bering Sea and in every community on the Panhandle from Skagway to Ketchikan. Towns there were in a unique position. They were isolated from each other but fairly well supplied with doctors and nurses. They tended their own, buried their own, and, perhaps strangely, recovered more rapidly than most. Governor Riggs requested and received medical help from Seattle, which may have contributed to the early flight of the disease.

The highest death rates occurred in the smaller communities to the north and west of the region. In the small Native village of Suitna on Cook Inlet, all but two of the 250 residents were ill by November 16. With everyone sick at once, there was no one to care for them, and help was eight days in arriving. By then most people were too ill to carry fuel to heat their homes or to prepare meals. The death toll was 29.

Kodiak Island fought the disease alone with no help from the outside for two months. In the population of 50 whites and 500

Aleuts, flu struck a third and 47 people died. Teller lost nearly half of its people; only 80 out of 150 survived. Corpses accumulated in cabins because no one was strong enough to drag them outside, and it was sometimes days before those well enough to manage their removal arrived. Bodies of friends and relatives were then stacked in the icy, snow-packed streets, where they lay frozen until the residents recovered and were able to arrange proper burials.

In a few communities where a respected leader took charge and insisted that no strangers be allowed in, the results were happier. In one Yukon mountain village, a teacher wrote, "Flu reached a point only 19 miles away, but halted there for lack of a medium on which to feed."

By mid-February 1919 the major wave of the flu had run its course, and quarantines in Alaska were lifted, except for the one in Skagway. In March 1919 there was a second wave of the disease, resulting in 40 new cases in Skagway and 15 in Cordova. In Fairbanks, two-thirds of the population was ill, but deaths were few and this wave was a pale sequel to its predecessor. Through the fall of 1918 and the spring of 1919, deaths in Alaska totalled 150 whites and nearly 2,000 Natives. As much as 8 percent of the Aboriginal population died.

On Canada's Labrador coast, the pandemic arrived only days earlier than it did in Alaska, and once again it came by sea. This time it was a supply boat that visited the area during mid-October, bringing with it news of the terrible flu and the flu itself. Records from the *Grenfell Mission*, a hospital ship that supplied services to the region, tell the story. Reverend Henry Gordon visited Cartwright on October 31. Only two weeks later, to his great surprise and horror, he found the settlement silent, not a soul in sight save a staggering man almost too sick to walk. He explained that the whole community had taken to their beds, struck with the illness only two days after the departure of the supply ship. Gordon visited the homes and found whole families prostrate. Only four of the 100 inhabitants of Cartwright were not ill. Within three days the reverend himself was too ill to help anyone, and a boy of 14 was the only one available to make coffins for the dead and dying. By the end of November one-quarter of the population was gone.

When Reverend Gordon recovered, he visited other communities to offer assistance. In one, he found 10 out of 26 people dead, still in their beds because everyone else was too sick to move them. He reported that one survivor, a woman of 72, had lived alone for nine days, with no fire and little food. All other members of the family had died and lay about her in the house. In every community, Reverend Gordon found similar situations. In one small settlement, three out of four families in one small settlement were all dead; in the fourth family, only the children had survived. At Okak, only 59 of more than 250 survived, and Gordon's group spent two weeks digging a hole 8 feet deep by 32 feet long, large enough to accommodate 114 bodies.

In one badly stricken community, the only survivor was an eight-year-old girl. As her family lay still around her, she had watched starving husky dogs eat their bodies. In another settlement, the stricken residents, with no soil deep enough to hold the bodies of the dead, weighed them down with rocks and dropped them into the sea from an overhanging bluff. It was all they could manage in their weakened condition.

The stories from these two widely separated areas of North America graphically illustrate the horrors experienced in the smallest and most isolated settlements when the Spanish Lady delivered her sentence of sickness and death.

IN THE WAKE
OF THE PANDEMIC

For 18 months the Spanish Lady went on a killing spree in North America, and then she stole away, leaving few clues as to where she originated or why she was fatal to so many. She touched every corner of the earth in her three years, leaving behind the worst death toll recorded in modern times. There are many estimates of the number of people who died—and they vary dramatically. They range as high as 40 to 50 million people worldwide, including 12 million in India alone. Among the estimates available are: 600,000 in Germany, 150,000 in England and Wales, 548,000 in the United States, and 50,000 in Canada. How many died in China and through most of Asia is anyone's guess.

In Canada, the largest number of casualties by far was in the more heavily populated provinces: Quebec, with 13,880 reported deaths, and Ontario with 8,705. The toll in Montreal was about 4,000, and in Toronto it was almost the same. In the other provinces, the death toll is estimated at about 1,400 in New Brunswick; in Prince Edward Island, 400; in Manitoba, 3,300; in Saskatchewan, 4,800; in Alberta, 4,300; and in British Columbia, more than 4,400. No figures are available for Nova Scotia, the Yukon, the Northwest Territories, Newfoundland, or Labrador, but thousands more died there.

Provincial Health Officer Dr. Young made it clear that the number of British Columbians who died in the pandemic was not known exactly, and other top medical men across the continent made similar admissions. In his annual report tabled in the Legislature in mid-1919, Young estimated that the flu took the lives of about one percent of the population (approximately 4,400 people). The provincial government had earlier given preliminary figures for deaths from October to December 1918 as 2,014. Young's report indicated an actual toll about twice that. The earlier figures apparently had not included many of the Aboriginal people who died.

The overall total for B.C. seemed high, but Young stated that in comparison with other areas "we were amongst the fortunate ones." Later figures compiled by major cities in North America showed that Vancouver had suffered one of the highest death rates: 795 victims, or 23.3 percent of every 1,000 cases. Winnipeg had 1021 deaths, or 16.7 percent of every 1,000 cases; New York, 27,362, or 14.4 percent per 1,000. Philadelphia headed the list with 14,198 deaths, or 24.7 percent per 1,000 cases.

The final figure for the number of deaths recorded in the larger area of the Lower Mainland was considerably more than 1,000, even if only based on Young's one percent of the population calculation. Underhill had kept close tabs on the city's cases and deaths and produced more accurate statistics than other nearby communities. He provided the number of deaths for Vancouver City proper as 618 from October 5 to December 31, 1918, and there were dozens more in the early months of 1919. The total number of cases reported in Vancouver to December 31 was 4,890, with the highest daily count of 1,304 cases in hospital on October 25. The worst 24-hour death toll was October 27, when 24 died.

One other assessment was made. Vancouver's mortality rate for the last three months of the year was 6.03 per 1,000 of population, with an interesting ethnic division, given that whites were by far the largest group. It showed: whites, 516, or 5.47 percent per 1,000; Chinese, 37, or 7.40 percent per 1,000; Japanese, 61, or 18.77 percent per 1,000; and Hindu, 4, or 15 percent per 1,000.

B.C.'s top medical man admitted in his report that the new strain of the disease "found us ill-prepared to meet the overwhelming calamity." The doctor said it could be concluded that about 30 percent of British Columbians had been affected, adding: "This no doubt will

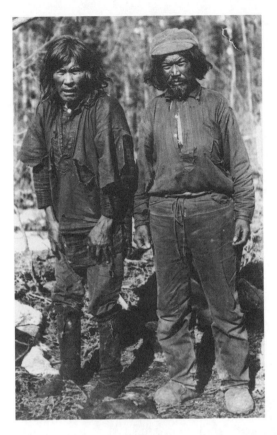

The flu seemed to hit Aboriginal people even harder than it did whites. St. Stephen's Anglican Church in Little Salmon, Yukon Territory, is pictured below as it was in 1913—the mission was abandoned when the local Little Salmon people were wiped out by the Spanish flu. Johnny Jack (left) and his father were two of the Little Salmon people who were decimated by the flu.

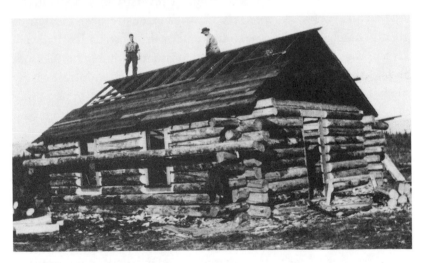

confer a certain degree of immunity." He stressed, however, that still "there is no vaccine against flu." Dr. Young paid tribute to his fellow citizens, lauding them for having acted nobly in their response to calls for assistance during the crisis. Along with all the tragedy, he reiterated, there had been one huge benefit: People appreciated the fact that greater personal and public hygiene was essential.

Military files provide a little more information on the flu's effects on Canada. Its records were superior to any kept by provincial health departments, particularly concerning the number of people hospitalized. From January 1 to October 31, 1918, among troops in Canada not yet overseas, there were 43,312 admissions to hospitals for various illnesses, with 852 deaths. Flu accounted for 23 percent of these. During the peak of the pandemic, it accounted for 49 percent. The number of cases and the death rate overseas were huge but harder to tabulate because of battlefield conditions. One report said that the flu claimed a total of 716 servicemen in Canada and 776 servicemen overseas during the period from September to December 1918, the months in which the disease was at its worst.

These statistics stood as the only record of the 1918 flu for many years, since little worthwhile analysis or research was done. One finely detailed book did eventually come out in 1976. It was written by Alfred W. Crosby and published by Greenwood Press under the title *Epidemic and Peace*. In 1989 Cambridge University Press reprinted it as *America's Forgotten Pandemic*. Crosby's extensive post-mortem is greatly enhanced by the case studies and wealth of statistics that were kept in the United States. He also records anecdotal material from around the world, and story after story contains reminiscences by survivors and witnesses that seem to vie with each other in plumbing the depths of sorrow, suffering, helplessness, and fear accompanying each pain-racked death. Every numbing account can be matched many times over.

Crosby's accounts and statistics on how the U.S. armed forces suffered are astonishing. The U.S. did not enter the war until 1917 and lost about 30,000 troops in action in one year, a terrible but still miniscule number compared with the other major nations involved. Sickness, he states, claimed more American soldiers than did shot and shell. "For every American soldier who died in battle or as a result of wounds or gas in World War One, 1.02 died of disease," he writes, adding that flu took the great majority.

At many army camps, the death toll was unbelievable. Across the country in mid-1918 there were many shoddily built hospitals that had been thrown up in a hurry. These turned into charnel houses as bodies piled up waiting to be buried, quickly rotting in the heat of summer. Camps were often beset by rats and other vermin. It did not take long for the situation to become critical, and within months, new rules and regulations in the American military were set out, covering everything from construction standards to hygiene and nutrition. Meanwhile, U.S. army doctors probed for causes of the Spanish flu without finding anything more than had been discovered in the civilian world.

After 1918: a new health department

The bottom line by 1919 was that there was no cure for the Spanish flu, little effective treatment, and even less hope of finding one. Britain's chief medical health officer, George Newman, had a particularly pessimistic outlook that came across quite clearly, even if couched in a typical stiff-upper-lip style. In his report submitted to Health Minister Christopher Addison after the pandemic, he wrote: "The prospect [of dealing with flu] is not hopeful but we must face it with equanimity and all the resourcefulness of the spirit of adventure and quest." He added that the world outlook on flu and further pestilence was indeed "gloomy," but a to-the-top-of-Everest spirit must prevail.

It was a situation that would prevail until enemies and allies alike had dealt with the war's aftermath. Their minds numbed by the terrible years of conflict and death, people the world over wanted desperately to forget the events of 1918 and put all the years of fear and suffering behind them. There had been too much sorrow for too long. Everyone needed to get on with life, and they did just that. On a national scale, Canada shared in a global need for massive spending on reconstruction and a new start after four years of neglect in which progress had been halted while funds were expended to fight the foe. There were new jobs to be found, massive rebuilding was essential, and new projects were ready and waiting to be undertaken. It would be many years before anyone studied in depth the flu's causes and effects, or the mistakes made in dealing with the worst pandemic of the 20th century.

There was one group, however, that found this approach impossible: the life-insurance companies. The Metropolitan Life Insurance Company in particular was in dire straits early in 1919, as it had paid death benefits in the U.S. and Canada for 83,000 people. Only because the company was so large was it able to weather the enormous payouts it was obliged to make.

Federal government ministers also could not forget the Spanish flu. The need for a coordinating medical body in Canada had become so blatantly obvious during the pandemic that every politician knew it was an issue that would dominate the next election unless something was done immediately. It was the one big issue that had to be addressed before getting on with business. It would be part of creating a new future for Canada.

Even prior to this fearful flu outbreak, there had been pressure from several sectors for a national health department to co-ordinate and foster preventative medicine and public health. Unfortunately, the establishment of such a body had always been thwarted by petty disagreements and arguments about infringements on provincial rights. Most of the complaints came from doctors who objected to the amount of time they would have to waste on all the paperwork that a new level of bureaucracy would entail. These objections all but disappeared when officials at all levels across the country realized the awful price the flu had exacted, and it became crystal-clear that many regions had little in the way of medical services. It was a situation that had to be remedied.

This point had been made in Parliament during the pandemic, and the common suffering of the population forced the issue. Objections suddenly evaporated and work began very quickly on preparing the final legislation to create a federal health department. The legislation was already drafted and, with unusual speed, the bill was introduced in the House on March 26, 1919, by Privy Council President H.W. Rowell. Debate was brief. Rowell stated that the new department would lead the drive to reduce Canada's high infant mortality rate and find cures for infectious diseases that caused so much sickness and death. The bill passed in the House of Commons on April 11—citizens of the time could not recall another debate in the House that went so smoothly and was resolved so rapidly—and Canada's federal health department was established, the forerunner to Health Canada. The creation of Canada's first national public health department was the most important development to come out of the pandemic.

The evolution of Canada's health-care system is a story in its own right, and today Health Canada faces even more challenges than its precursor did when it was first established. Now the challenges include not only responding to public need, but also controlling the enormous expenditures being made at federal and provincial levels to maintain a system that is evolving at unbelievable speed—a system that shows no signs of becoming any less important or less costly in the future. The SARS crisis of 2003 prompted the then-federal health minister Anne McLellan to pledge the government to "rebuild and enhance" the whole system. Her immediate successor, Pierre Pettigrew, has not indicated whether or not he agrees.

Today any flu epidemic or pandemic falls under the purview of the Centre for Infectious Disease Prevention and Control, a part of Canada's Health and Welfare Department in Ottawa, and each province has its own centre for disease control. Interviewed in late 2003 for this book, Dr. Theresa Tam, chief of immunization and respiratory infections for Health Canada, said that before the SARS epidemic, Canada had a flu-watch system that was regarded in medical circles both in Canada and the U.S. as one of the best. It was designed to collect and provide full information about flu outbreaks across the country on a continuing basis, to help scientists identify the many strains of viruses that arrive each year. The watch is a co-operative effort between the federal and provincial governments, laboratories, the College of Family Physicians of Canada, and other organizations. But as the fast-moving and mysterious SARS strain illustrated and as the SARS Advisory Committee appointed at the time to investigate the disease emphasized, more funds and resources are necessary to meet a new and very real challenge.

Dr. Tam said the federal government began spending more on flu research in the late 1990s, and that much of the money went into providing millions of flu shots and into research to find more effective vaccines. She added that stepping up anti-viral production in Canada to meet our own needs is being pursued in order to reduce our reliance on imports, which will not be available in the event of a true pandemic. We always face the reality that a new flu vaccine takes four to six months to develop. It cannot be purchased in advance and stored. Its creation utilizes millions of eggs, and its shelf life is limited.

Dr. Tam's monitoring and identification data are passed on to the World Health Organization, an international group with centres in London, England; Tokyo, Japan; Melbourne, Australia; and, the largest centre of all, Atlanta, Georgia. In 1918 the Spanish flu virus remained unknown and unidentified. Today, whenever there is a need to identify a new virus, it is a worldwide collaboration within the World Health Organization. Much work for the cause also goes on in laboratories and universities in other countries, including Canada. The WHO tracks disease at the international level and can move quickly to institute travel bans and protective procedures.

At a humbler level, in many countries an annual flu shot for children and the elderly has become a recommended procedure. It is not a cure, but an immunization that aims to lessen the serious effects of the disease.

The research effort

Over the years medical experts looked at the many questions arising from the 1918 pandemic, as well as from other fast-spreading diseases. By the 1930s they had identified viruses as the source of most flu epidemics, but other questions remained. What was the difference between the common cold and influenza? What was different about the Spanish flu pandemic, and why did some people develop the pneumonia that was so often fatal? Some doctors have postulated that the 1918 outbreak should not be considered a flu pandemic, but a pneumonic one, since pneumonia was often the ultimate killer.

A great multitude of other contradictory questions were raised. Was Spanish flu different, or was there a common factor? Why were young children and the elderly often spared? The most puzzling fact was that the majority of victims were young and seemingly healthy adults. Because the elderly were more often than not among the lucky ones, it was assumed that some of them had developed immunity during their exposure to the 1889–1890 flu.

It was natural to look at the war for a cause of the pandemic. There were those who were firmly convinced that the Germans had something to do with it because of their initial use of poison gas. Could they also have used a flu virus as a weapon? If they had, it had certainly backfired: Germany suffered more than many other countries during the pandemic. The zealots could not be convinced and they were loud and persistent. One contended that the outbreak should not be called the Spanish flu, but rather "the German Plague." Speculation about the cause of the flu abounded, with theories ranging from the rational to the totally bizarre, such as extraterrestrial involvement.

Scientists did look to the war for causes, but found only more conundrums. The squalor and starvation created by rampaging armies has always been a breeding ground for infectious diseases and sickness. Some scientists were convinced that the deprivations of war had produced the pandemic, but this was not the case. Extensive studies revealed that the number of cases and deaths was not much different in the war-ravaged countries than it was in those with no battlefields on their lands. Canada and the United States were battered by the pandemic even though the war was not fought on their home ground. There had been no fighting or dislocation in Great Britain, but it also suffered very badly. There were no answers.

As the years went by, some scientists became more concerned about the phenomenon of the flu and began to take a new look at it. More money and resources were devoted to the hunt. Centres were established in several countries, modern laboratories were funded, and there developed a new generation of scientific specialists who were devoted to infectious-disease identification and control. They were intrigued by the flu and all its mysteries and were prepared to engage in years of probing and experimenting. Results throughout the 1920s produced both optimism and bleak despair as great efforts led nowhere, but gradually advances in knowledge were made.

In 1921, a team of eminent American scientists threw out years of research done to support Pfeiffer's claim that his bacillus was the main cause of flu—they had decided that it was not. Four decades later, one of those scientists said they had been 100 percent wrong

185

to throw out that work. Such is the course of research, and much has continued based on Pfeiffer's discovery.

Some of this work involved Canadian researchers. Using identical techniques, two groups, one in Canada and one in England, came up with different results. The Canadians found Pfeiffer's bacillus in 24 percent of the Toronto cases they checked, while a British group found it in almost all of the cases it studied. Similar discrepancies were found around the world. Scientists wondered if they had successfully demonstrated a link between the bacillus and the Spanish flu when they transferred a specimen obtained from a child with flu and pneumonia to white laboratory mice, and then from the mice to monkeys. Some of the monkeys died with what appeared to be the same lung conditions as the Spanish flu victims had. But the tests were inconclusive and subject to wide interpretation. Nonetheless, experiments continued in the U.S., Britain, Canada, Japan, Germany, France, and every other country with advanced medical facilities.

Unexpectedly, there was a big break for the dogs of the world when a Harvard University bacteriologist suggested in the early 1920s that whoever found the answer to canine distemper, a major deadly killer in the canine world, would also advance the cause of finding a flu cure. The bacteriologist gained support because there were others who had recognized the similarity between distemper and the flu, although they definitely were not the same. The dog-loving British were anxious to beat distemper, and the Medical Research Council was given money to probe the question. Dog-lovers in Canada, other parts of the British Empire, and in the U.S. added money to the research funding. It paid off: In 1926, G.W. Dunkin and Patrick Playfair Laidlaw, researchers working at England's Mill Hill laboratories, tracked down and identified the guilty virus. A distemper vaccine was soon developed that today continues to offer protection to the doggie world. The work also added to humankind's knowledge about the flu and advanced the fight against it.

There was another and, for the world's human population, larger breakthrough a few years later. In the First World War, many soldiers had died from wound infections; Alexander Fleming was horrified by the deaths he saw while serving with the British army. After the war he began to look for something that would halt such infections and, at the same time, combat the influenza virus.

Fleming sought to produce a pure culture of Pfeiffer's bacillus. While working in his lab, he inadvertently left some culture plates of *staphylococci* open to contamination. Later, Fleming found them all dead except for Pfeiffer's bacillus, resulting in one of the great breakthroughs for humankind. The *cocci* had been wiped out by a penicillin mould that had formed. Penicillin became the wonder antibiotic that has cured infections the world over. Fleming's work, for which he gained international acclaim and honours, again helped advance the scientific war against flu, but did not provide the information he had been seeking originally.

In 1933, following a flu outbreak in Britain, scientists Wilson Smith, C.H. Andrewes, and P.P. Laidlaw decided to try some experiments using the ferret, a relative of the weasel, because of its susceptibility to distemper. Laidlaw had previously been involved in research that showed that this species almost always died on contracting distemper. After complicated tests at the Mill Hill laboratories, and the transmission of what they believed to be flu from one ferret to another, they finally announced that they had isolated the infective agent of flu that caused the disease.

Acclaim followed, along with the kind of debate and scepticism that meets every new development in the scientific world. It remained clear that much had still to be done, although among the doubters there was generally an admission that the trio had gone beyond Pfeiffer's work. Even Laidlaw was cautious in remarks made some two years after their success. He stated: "I believe that it is now being gradually proved that the primary infective agent in epidemic flu is a filterable virus." At the same time, he acknowledged that there were those who maintained that Pfeiffer's bacillus was the prime cause of flu and the complications it produced. Laidlaw was correct.

Research continued, although by the mid-1930s medical science was increasingly directed toward the prospects of another war and the problems that new weapons and new types of wounds and injuries could bring. Only 21 years after the guns stopped in Flanders, the events of 1939 ushered in another act of global slaughter.

187

During the Second World War there were minor attacks of flu and other infectious diseases around the globe. One of the episodes reported in Canada took place in 1942, at Cambridge Bay in the Arctic, where 15 Eskimos died. Many others were sick, but the community's isolation prevented any spread of the illness. Studies were later completed to determine whether any disease developed as a result of the Second World War, but despite the misery, destruction, and mass movement of people under the direst conditions, which produced much sickness, there was no pandemic or flu comparable to that of 1918.

Since the 1950s flu viruses have been classified according to the proteins found on their outer skins. One is called haemagglutinin (H), and the other neuraminidase (N). To date, scientists have identified flu strains with 15 different forms of H and with nine different variations of N. Viruses are now identified by labels such as H1N1, H2N2, and so on.

One avenue of research in recent times has led scientists on a bizarre hunt to find victims of the Spanish flu. They have been searching for lung tissue or other organ parts from victims of the 1918 pandemic in the hope of determining exactly what dreadful strain it was. The discovery of still-complete bodies from Franklin's fatal mid-1800s expedition to the Canadian Arctic helped intensify interest. The sailors who died in the expedition to find the Northwest Passage had been buried in permafrost, and their frozen bodies were in fairly good condition when they were discovered more than 100 years later. Thus the question was, where might 1918 victims have been buried in similar conditions?

There was a Canadian-inspired attempt to find tissue from flu victims who had died on barren, lonely Spitzbergen Island, north of Norway in the Arctic Ocean. Spitzbergen Island, the largest of the Svarlbard group, is a forbidding place, a four-and-a-half-hour plane flight from Oslo, with a stopover at Tromso. Basically, it is a treeless, barren lump of rock with a fearsome climate. The first explorers recorded visiting it more than 500 years ago. Much later it became a centre for whaling and mining. Seven young Norwegian men died there in 1918 after going there to work in the coal mines, bringing the Spanish flu with them.

Kirsty Duncan, an eager young Toronto woman with a degree in geography, became interested in the Spanish flu after reading Alfred Crosby's book in the early '90s. She was interested in how climatic change and other events throughout the world could affect health. She became intrigued with the idea that if human tissue could be recovered from the Franklin victims, then the bodies of the young Norwegians buried on Spitzbergen might still contain the Spanish flu virus.

Duncan knew of a small 1951 expedition to Alaska by Johan Hultin, who believed the Spanish flu virus could be found in the remains of northern 1918 victims. At Teller Mission, in the Seward Peninsula in Alaska where thousands of Natives perished, researchers opened a mass grave and collected samples of lungs, kidneys, and other organs. Back in their Iowa laboratories, the Hultin-expedition scientists were able to revive *pneumococci* bacteria and Pfeiffer's bacillus, but the killer flu virus remained unidentified.

Duncan persuaded various organizations to mount a campaign for her search. In 1998, her team recovered bodies from Spitzbergen graves, but the young men had not been buried deep enough to be preserved in permafrost, and apart from bones and non-lung tissue, nothing was recovered that could help isolate the Spanish Lady.

While Duncan, who seemed to alienate many of the scientists she encountered, sought more funds and publicity, Hultin remounted a quieter expedition to Alaska. This time he was successful in isolating the virus, and he brought samples to fellow scientist Jeffrey Taubenberger. Extraction of RNA from lung tissue of 1918 flu victims enabled scientists to sequence the influenza virus genome for the first time. The research indicated that the virus might not have come directly from a bird but was most probably associated with another host. Sequencing of more avian H1 strains and more research into possible intermediate hosts for the 1918 pandemic, such as swine, are now being done. There is an urgent need to identify the virus, for until its true origins are understood, another similar pandemic could go undetected for some time.

The tireless hunt for one of the world's most lethal viruses never stops. Recently, virologist Dr. John Oxford reported that a team from St. Bartholomew's Hospital in London, England, hoped to get valuable information from the body of Phyllis Burns, who died of the flu in October 1918 at age 20. Scientists learned that she had been buried in a lead coffin and entombed in a brick vault; they thought such conditions could have preserved her body sufficiently for organ tissue to be found. At the time of this writing, the team was seeking relatives of Burns for permission to exhume her. Oxford stated that it was a "scientific endeavour that has a good chance of producing information with the potential to save many lives." There seems always to be more information, if not yet anything truly conclusive.

The scientific advances in viral identification have led to legal concerns. Lawyers may have smiled in 2003 when a report contended that colds, flu, and other infections can now be traced back to the people who passed them on. David Hillis, a scientist from the University of Texas, where this research has been carried out, said: "In principle this type of analysis could be conducted with any virus, but I hope we don't degenerate into people blaming each other for passing on colds." Some commentators hoped that this new tracing system didn't throw open the doors to an avalanche of lawsuits and litigation, based on evidence that "he gave it to me." However, this is a minor worry compared to that of the viruses themselves.

Modern flu outbreaks

Throughout the 1940s, Canada dealt with many flu outbreaks, most of them fairly localized and not of major proportions, although the cumulative toll was enough to provide a constant spur to the hunt for a cure.

The country was less fortunate in the 1950s. In 1951 Ottawa set up a flu information centre when an epidemic claimed hundreds of lives in Britain, and there were fears it might reach across the Atlantic. The outbreak seemed to originate in Scandinavia, where there were many deaths. In an effort to prevent it from coming to Canada, Trans-Canada Air Lines, forerunner of Air Canada, announced that all people flying from England to Canada would be medically inspected before take-off and again after landing. None of the fliers were found to be sick on arrival, although it was possible some were in the very early stages of infection. This was when trans-Atlantic flights took much longer than today's jets. It also was a time when most people crossed the ocean by liner and any illness was detectable during the much longer sea voyage.

Despite the safeguards, the 1950s flu wasn't stopped, although it was much less severe than the 1918 variety. New Brunswick was hardest hit: a total of 102 people died between November 1950 and March 31, 1951. There were other deaths across Canada, but the numbers were not staggering. B.C. was lucky—only a minor outbreak was experienced. Provincial authorities, however, found it necessary to counteract quickly a frightening report that could have produced panic. Nobody knew where it originated, but one rather flamboyant reporter contended some 20,000 people had contracted the disease in B.C.'s central Okanagan Valley. Government officials just as rapidly pointed out that there was barely that number of people in the entire area, and only a handful of them had the sniffles.

In 1953 Canada, in co-operation with the World Health Organization, distributed 7,000 test doses of a new flu vaccine produced by Connaught Laboratories in Toronto. It was given to groups of hospital employees, members of the armed forces, and industrial workers. Unfortunately, results were inconclusive and the value of the vaccine remained undetermined.

In 1966, A.A. Larsen, head of B.C.'s division of epidemiology, reported to Ottawa that a severe local outbreak had taken 106 lives between February and April. He emphasized that provincial experts had been unable to identify the strain. Three years later he reported another minor outbreak in the Interior, but it was a much milder form.

A million people died in 1957 from an Asian flu identified as H1N1. The Hong Kong flu of 1968 was H3N2, and the Hong Kong virus of 1997 was identified as H5N1. Both were chicken viruses passed to humans. Most virologists now believe that when a virus jumps species, it may not initially be serious, but that given time it will mutate. Once its genes have been reshuffled, it will adapt to its new human host, becoming readily transmittable and sometimes, although not always, more deadly. They also agree that any H5 virus is extremely dangerous.

In his book first published in England in 1999 as *Catching Cold* and a year later in the U.S. as *The Devil's Flu,* author Pete Davies describes the 1997 Hong Kong flu. Nearly 7,000 birds died from a viral infection that began in March 1997. By May it had spread to humans, and 12-year-old boy died. This led to one of the most frightening outbreaks of flu since the 1918 pandemic, carrying within it the potential to kill millions upon millions of people. Well aware of the possibility of an impending tragedy if the virus swept through crowded Hong Kong, health officials took drastic, swift action.

The virus was isolated by the Department of Agriculture and Fisheries and identified as a dangerous strain. The information about the virus was passed to Kenneth Shortridge, chair of microbiology at Hong Kong's university. Within days, working around the clock, he confirmed the H5N1 virus and ordered the destruction of all chickens in the territory. This H5 virus was the ultimate challenge for Hong Kong's public health officer, Paul Saw.

Shortridge informed the World Health Organization's centre in Atlanta and asked the man in charge, Ron Webster, if killing all the chickens was the right thing to do. Webster's response was, "If they hadn't been killed, I would predict that you and I wouldn't be sitting here talking now, because one of us would be dead." In 1983, the U.S. Department of Agriculture had ordered the slaughter of 20 million chickens following a similar outbreak in Pennsylvania.

Shortridge, originally from Queensland, Australia, has lived in Hong Kong for 25 years and argues that southern China—in fact, all of southeast Asia—is the source of many new and dangerous viruses. Other scientists also said in 1997 that the Hong Kong chicken flu outbreak bolstered their view of this region as a flu "epicentre," caused by people living in close proximity with fowl, swine, and other livestock in crowded dwellings and markets in small villages and towns that sell live animals and birds.

New viruses and SARS

In a masterful understatement, one medical expert wrote in the year 2000 that the behaviour of the flu "borders on the miraculous and fills us with wonder and astonishment." He agreed that today's medical advances make the world better prepared to fight the disease, but the new strains of the virus that keep appearing need new vaccines, and humankind is constantly playing catch-up, trying desperately to prevent localized epidemics from becoming pandemics.

The importance of the World Health Organization has been proven many times over, but at no time was it more evident than in 2003. As Elinor Levy and Mark Fischetti explained in *The New Killer Diseases*:

> When WHO contacts from around the world met in Geneva on Saturday, March 15, 2003, they brought with them as much local intelligence as they could. Their reports revealed that this new mystery illness was highly contagious—it was infecting so many people so quickly in Hong Kong, Singapore, Vietnam, and Toronto that it must be spreading by simple close contact—people coughing or sneezing on one another. And it had hopped continents so easily that people must remain contagious for some time, meaning travelers could spread the pathogen far and wide. WHO officials issued a statement right after the meeting ended saying that the illness was a 'worldwide health threat'—a pronouncement WHO had never made before at the outset of any new disease, not even AIDS.

The establishment of the Michael Smith Genome Sciences Centre in Vancouver put Canada in the forefront when it came to identifying the SARS virus, which invaded both Toronto and Vancouver. The centre and three of its scientists, Dr. Marco Marra, Dr. Caroline Astell, and Dr. Steven Jones, were the first to post the blueprint of the virus on the Internet. Atlanta was second, and it congratulated the Vancouver scientists on their achievement.

According to Dr. Earl Brown, a virologist at the University of Ottawa who has devoted his life to the study of viruses and why some become mass killers, ominous similarities exist between SARS and the 1918 flu. Brown claims that SARS was actually deadlier than the

1918 flu virus because it killed 4 percent of its victims whereas the 1918 variety killed only 2.5 percent. Nevertheless, the real figures were 44 SARS deaths compared to 50,000 in 1918.

SARS, like the Spanish flu, did not follow the typical pattern of a viral outbreak, starting strong and ugly and weakening quickly. Brown contends that early detection is key to dealing with a SARS outbreak and points out the differences between the controls used in Vancouver and Toronto. Early action by Vancouver produced isolation and barrier nursing techniques to protect its health-care workers. In Toronto, there was no early detection, resulting in extensive infection of medical personnel and their families. Brown says that during the six weeks when the disease was at its peak, Toronto had 150 cases and a stunning 15 percent death rate, while Vancouver had only four cases and no deaths. SARS started strong, and it remains unclear whether it weakened or merely ran out of people to infect.

The federal government set up a SARS National Advisory Committee in May 2003, soon after the disease hit Canada. The committee quickly conducted an inquiry, and its report in October 2003 said that the SARS experience illustrates that even today "Canada is not adequately prepared to deal with a true pandemic."

The committee was highly critical of all levels of government: "SARS is simply the latest in a series of recent bellwethers for the fragile state of Canada's federal/provincial/municipal/ public health systems. The pattern is now familiar. Public health is taken for granted until disease outbreaks occur, whereupon a brief flurry of lip service leads to minimal investments and little real change in public health infrastructures or priorities. This cycle must end."

It was fortunate that the 2003 outbreak was "primarily centred in a major urban area [Toronto] with unparalleled health-care resources," the report contended. But it stressed that the lessons learned point to the real needs of the future in a world where diseases move at jet speed. Improvements that the country needs include a better surveillance mechanism, better co-ordination among the various levels of government and institutions for outbreak containment, improved public communications strategies, and major increases in expert human resources.

For years Dr. Allison McGeer, one of Canada's leading communicable-disease experts, has lobbied for fully enclosed rooms in emergency departments and more space between patients' beds in order to better control the spread of pathogens. She is currently a physician at Toronto's Mount Sinai Hospital. Says Dr. McGeer: "It took all of my department's efforts to get a single isolation room in our emergency department at Mount Sinai." It is anticipated that in the future, hospital designers will take more seriously McGeer's pleas for dealing with infectious disease issues. After all, one of the reasons for Vancouver's control of SARS was the speed with which patients were isolated.

As always, the major problem is money. The committee recommended that Ottawa alone pump another $700 million a year into the public health system by 2007 and create a new Canadian Agency for Public Health, headed by a chief public health officer. It seems odd that 85 years after Canada's first medical health department was created, there is a call for a new chief public health office.

Dr. Robert C. Burnham, medical director of the B.C. Centre for Disease Control in Vancouver, was a member of the SARS Advisory Committee. He said that his was the only public health agency of its kind in Canada, and expected that it would play a major role in establishing a new federal public health agency. Burnham said that the creation of such an organization would be a major step in meeting the increasing challenges to public health. He added that B.C.'s SARS experience was minor, and while "luck" played a part in its containment, it was obvious that organizations such as his had an important role to play in surveillance and notification. The B.C. Centre has state-of-the-art facilities, built in 1997, and receives $70 million annually from the provincial government, $30 million going to vaccines for preventable childhood diseases.

One thing is evident: The suddenness of the SARS attack, with only the policy of isolating victims helping to hold down the fatality rate, makes the public and governments more aware of the dangers of a new pandemic.

In January 2004, many of the southeast Asian countries— Vietnam, Thailand, and Korea, to name a few—experienced an outbreak of avian flu. It was fatal in virtually all of the chickens it infected; in January alone, it killed more than one million birds. Numerous children also died. The outbreak in Vietnam prompted Klaus Stohr, project leader of the WHO's global influenza program, to say, "The ingredients are there that the pandemic can occur."

An outbreak of avian flu in the Fraser Valley of B.C. in the spring of 2004 resulted in authorities ordering the extermination of all fowl in the region. Fortunately, the virus was an H7 and not an H5.

In Vancouver, Dr. Danuta Skowronski, an influenza specialist at the B.C. Centre for Disease Control, commented, "The more times that there are outbreaks amongst poultry and the more times that there are human exposures and human cases of H5N1, the more opportunities there are for this flu virus to mutate to the point where it is well adapted for human-to-human transmission."

As doctors warn that the next flu pandemic could make SARS seem trivial, Health Canada has developed a new national influenza response plan. It has been in the works since 1988. There is, unfortunately, at least one huge roadblock: Nothing can accelerate the time it takes to develop a new vaccine, a period of four to six months. A stockpile of anti-viral drugs would be a help, and that is something no country, including Canada, has even begun to do. Dr. Skowronski points out that up to 50,000 Canadians could become ill with influenza at once, making it critical for the country to have large supplies of general anti-viral drugs. Health Canada is working with Shire Biologics of Saint-Foy, Quebec, to ensure that eight million doses of vaccine could be produced each month. A new class of anti-viral drugs called neuraminidase inhibitors targets the surface molecules of the flu viruses, shortening the duration of the flu, and another drug, Tamiflu, has the potential to reduce the risk of transmission between close contacts by 80 to 90 percent. Drug manufacturer Roche Laboratories has been negotiating with Health Canada to produce 600,000 doses of Tamiflu, enough to treat 60,000 people. Having supplies on hand could make a huge difference, but that won't happen in the short term, and the plan estimates that between 4.5 and 10.5 million people would be infected during a pandemic, leaving the country woefully short of supplies.

A worrisome complication developed from the viruses of early 2004. The vaccines designed to guard against them are usually grown and cultured in eggs, but the new deadly Asian strains that kill 100 percent of the infected birds also kill the eggs, so different methods of developing effective treatments against specific flu strains must be found.

"The smaller pandemics in 1957 and 1968 involved influenza strains derived from birds, and then there was the 1997 one," said Dr. Donald Low, chief of microbiology at Toronto's University Health Network and Mount Sinai Hospital. It's an alarming trend: "What's going on now in Asia is very disconcerting because what we're watching here is the evolution of this virus to a stage at which it would be the next pandemic."

The disturbing increase in viruses and the emergence of superbugs that are immune to antibiotics have sparked scientists to warn that more pathogens are infecting more people faster than ever before. About a million people in North America are infected each year with drug-resistant bacteria in hospitals, and 20,000 to 80,000 of these people die. When the rise in the number of bacteria immune to antibiotics and the increase in viruses and virus mutations are considered together, they pose a frightening picture for the future of the world. Norwalk disease, which hundreds of cruiseship passengers have come down with since the year 2000, and the waves of West Nile Virus in Ontario and Saskatchewan in 2003 are examples of new viral infections.

In late 2003, Dr. Robert G. Webster of St. Jude Children's Research Hospital in Memphis, Tennessee, was prompted to make a disturbing statement: "We don't even know they're [viruses] there until we disturb them. SARS is probably just a gentle breeze of what one of these big ones is going to do some day. There are thousands—maybe even millions—of viruses out there." They have only one thing in common: Animals pass them to humans.

Since the outbreak of SARS, a group of Asian scientists studying the wild-animal markets in China has found a corona virus like the one believed to have caused the 2003 outbreak, but it now has about 50 mutations in its RNA. Like the flu virus, a SARS corona virus tends to mutate steadily. Count the mutations, geneticists say, and you can figure out how far removed this new virus is from its ancestor. To date, the virus has been found in civets, dogs, and a ferret, as well as in birds and reptiles.

Elinor Levy and Mark Fischetti also point out:

The outbreak of SARS, the emergence of super-pathogens, and the increase in commingling of chronic infections all drive home just how complex a fight we must wage. We are in the midst of an evolutionary war against microbes that have proven more sophisticated and multi-talented than we could ever have expected. We cannot underestimate how serious the struggle is. It's obvious that our bodies alone are unable to outwit many pathogens. Now our drugs are failing as well. If we don't step up our efforts to strengthen our defences, the microbes might actually win in the long run. Unless we mobilize our resources more effectively, the risk is too high that there will be widespread suffering as well as social and economic disruption.

What all of these scientists fear most is a strain of influenza that has never before been seen in humans, a strain for which the only treatment available is isolation. It would break from nature anywhere and develop the ability to spread not just from animals to humans, but from human to human as well. No one would have immunity, so it would leap unchecked around the world. Health Canada estimates that 9,000 to 51,000 Canadians could die in the next pandemic if a vaccine is not available. And almost everyone studying the whole issue agrees that a pandemic is almost inevitable, and it may not be very far off.

Flu—always with us

Minor outbreaks of flu have become a fact of life for much of the world's population. While they are generally not too serious, they continue to bring discomfort, economic costs, and loss of life every year. They've become accepted as a vicissitude of winter, something one can't do much about.

In Canada, despite annual flu shots for an increasing number of Canadians, flu in one form or another is always with us. As Dr. John Blatherwick states:

For the first 15 years I was MHO in Vancouver,
I always explained that the influenza that we
would receive the next year was the influenza
circulating in Asia in the January/February of the
present year. Influenza would then arrive in British
Columbia usually in the week of Christmas after
first appearing in Alberta one week earlier. The
cases would climb throughout January and peak
in the February/early March period and then drop
off. In April we would see a small bump in cases as
Influenza B appeared.

There were five straight years when that was exactly what
happened, says Dr. Blatherwick:

And then the last three years—virtually no disease
in December—very light in early January—peak
in February/early March and no bump in April.
While the peak of the infections the last three years
was as bad as in previous years, the overall season
was greatly shortened and thus the number of
people affected was greatly diminished. Is vaccine
playing a part? Maybe! Has the influenza (current
strain) lessened in infectiousness? Maybe! What
has remained interesting is that the influenza seen
in North America has remained the strain seen the
year earlier in Asia. With air travel between Asia
and North America, one would think that the virus
circulating in Asia would appear at almost the same
time in North America, but it doesn't show up until
the next respiratory season. Odd!
    Also, influenza virus drifts each year. So when
you deal with an H3 N2 virus, it chains slightly
each year. However, pandemics occur when there is
a shift in the virus and one of the H or N actually
changes. There were three major shifts in the 20th
century—1918, probably, 1957, and 1968.

Influenza B, which seems to always be around, is milder than Influenza A. Immunization provides about 70 percent protection against B influenza if taken each year and it is because of the 'drift' that it has to be a new vaccine each year.

The flu virus in one of its many forms still claims up to 1,400 lives a year across the country. As of 2004, health authorities in B.C. were giving more than 900,000 free flu shots annually, and because of new threats of serious bouts of flu, that number was likely to increase. Dr. Ian Gemmill, chairman of the Canadian Coalition for Influenza Immunization, said flu shots "are the best, longest lasting, safest and most effective way to prevent influenza." Gemmill said shots prevent sickness in 70 to 90 percent of vaccinated adults when there is a good match of the vaccine to the strain that is present.

But the key problem is matching the strain to the vaccine. The headline in one B.C. newspaper of December 20, 2003, read: "Next Big B.C. Flu Outbreak Could Kill 6,800." The statement was attributed to Dr. Shaun Peck, deputy provincial health officer, who said, "A devastating flu outbreak that would make one in every two British Columbians sick and kill as many as 6,800 people could hit the province within the next five to ten years." It would be a pandemic, he said, because the outbreak would be of new virus and it takes six months to develop an effective vaccine. He added that there is now a pandemic influenza preparedness plan in place that will be followed when the outbreak hits B.C. It is the same procedure that was used when SARS arrived.

AFTERWORD

When the Spanish Lady crept away in 1919, those who played key roles resumed their usual busy lives, although the experiences, the crises, and the drama of the preceding months would live with them forever.

Dr. Young continued as an advocate for improved public health in B.C. He oversaw the creation of the University of B.C.'s faculty of nursing, recommended by Dr. McEachern in the fall of 1918 when he called for a period of formal training for student nurses before they began to work in hospital wards.

Education was a high priority for Dr. Young, who continued to receive accolades for his role in the creation and development of UBC. Earlier, while he was a politician, he had prepared the legislation to create the endowment lands at the tip of Point Grey as a site for the educational institution, and in 1907, when the legislature established the university, he wrote its constitution. When the move was made from the King Edward campus, which played such a prominent role during the pandemic, to the new campus at Point Grey in 1925, Dr. Young was hailed as "the father of the university." During the formal opening ceremonies, it was stated that both UBC and the expanded Essondale mental hospital were monuments to him "in brick and stone."

Dr. Young died at Victoria's Royal Jubilee Hospital on October 24, 1940, a few days after being admitted with heart problems. The following April, his 40 years of contributions and service to the province and its people were recognized in tributes from far and wide, and his ashes were scattered on the waters of Bubbins Bay at Hernando Island, where he had spent many happy summers.

Dr. McEachern became the president of the B.C. Hospital Association and president of the Public Health and Welfare Association of Greater Vancouver. He left VGH in 1922 and for a year was director general of the Victorian Order of Nurses for Canada. McEachern moved on to the United States and became an associate director of the American College of Surgeons; later, he was a director of professional relations of the American Hospital Association. McEachern was also an associate professor in the school of medicine at Chicago's Northwestern University. He established a reputation as one of North America's top professionals in the field of operating and managing hospitals, receiving many international awards for his work. He died in Chicago in 1956.

Mayor Gale left Vancouver and B.C. in the 1920s and returned to his hometown, Montreal, where he went back into private business. He was prominent in industrial production and the demands of war work after 1939. He died there in 1950.

Dr. Fred Underhill remained the indefatigable watchdog of Vancouver's health, continuing to push the ideas he had espoused when he first took on the job in 1904. He was admired and respected by nearly everyone and feared by those who transgressed the city bylaws that pertained to hygiene. There was no escape from his scrutiny. He was frustrated by the lack of public funds available when money became tight following the 1929 market collapse and Vancouver was faced by the Great Depression that ran well into the '30s. Equipment broke down and there was nothing to replace it; things he wanted to do remained undone; every scarce dollar was stretched to the limit in trying to care for the destitute and the children of the unemployed. Things were not the way he wanted them, but publicly, he never damned the present nor feared the future.

He was into his 70s, still dealing with the difficulties of the times, when he finally laid down his stethoscope in 1930. Many felt the city suffered a great loss. They were disappointed that little was done to honour the man who unstintingly gave so much of himself to his beloved adopted Vancouver. Well-wishers stated that Dr. Underhill had rendered "body and soul" to the city, and there were countless witnesses to the excellence and worth of his work, colleagues and friends from all walks of life. Their admiration for the doctor and their anger at the absence of a full and formal expression of appreciation from the city fathers were made abundantly clear in this testimonial, reported in the press:

> We feel that it is not enough that he should be allowed to go from the post which he so ably and conscientiously filled, without a word of gratitude and regret. Very little notice seems to have been taken by anyone of the fact that Vancouver is losing one of its ablest and most faithful servants, a man who for many years has been the guardian of our public health.
>
> It was his duty, of course, and he was paid to do it, although the less said about the latter the better. When one considers the miserable salary that was all this city could afford to pay to a man who for 30 years has filled one of the most important offices in its service, one feels rather ashamed. Still, he was paid a salary. Yet we feel this does not quite discharge the debt that Vancouver owes to Dr. Underhill. His was a particularly difficult and thankless task. Blame in plenty would have been his share, if owing to carelessness or neglect on his part, any great disaster had occurred. Yet when he did his duty, and, in spite of themselves, when he protected the citizens against infectious diseases, against epidemics, against impure milk and bad sanitary conditions, all too frequently he was attacked and opposed bitterly, and all too seldom received the support and backing that should have been given him. But none of this prevented him from doing his duty.
>
> Patiently, courageously, but courteously withal, he did what he knew should be done, and insisted

on those in authority doing the right thing. No easy job for any man, but he did it exceedingly well, and Vancouver today with its pure milk, its pure water, its well-kept food stores, and its comparative freedom from slums and disease traps, may thank Dr. Underhill for its blessings along these lines. Handicapped by lack of funds, by lack of staff, and by public apathy he never gave up the fight against dirt and disease and in his quiet unspectacular way, he achieved great victories.

Always courteous and gentle, he could yet be firm and insistent, and could even flame into righteous indignation. To all who knew him, it was a pleasure and an inspiration to have dealings with him, and one never failed to secure from him the fullest consideration, the most sincere and honest response, for he never attempted to dodge an issue put squarely to him. All too often he was unable to do what he would like, or wanted to do, but he gave his reasons frankly and candidly, and did the very best he could.

So we are sorry, very sorry, to see him go, and we feel that we should say so. We feel too, that the medical profession of this city should pay a tribute, a sincere and thankful tribute, to this man who has done so much honour to his profession, and been loyal to its very best traditions.

It would be most fitting that we should make some formal acknowledgement to Dr. Underhill of the esteem in which we hold him, and of the regret with which we see him leave the service of the city.

He has, we hope, many years of happy and peaceful life ahead of him, and we find it in us to envy the satisfaction and the peace of mind with which he can face these years. We wish him long life, and happiness and we say to him, "Well done!"

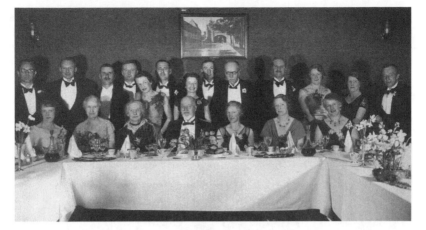

Frederick and Beatrice in 1935, after 50 years of marriage, are shown here surrounded by their children, sons-in-law, and daughters-in-law.

Dr. Fred Underhill had lived a long life, but his retirement was short. On April 17, 1936, after a fairly long illness, he died in Vancouver General Hospital, surrounded by members of his large, extended family. He was survived by sons Clare, James Theodore, William, John, and Richard, and by daughters Mrs. Harold Dyer of North Vancouver, Mrs. M.H. Vernon of Ottawa, Mrs. W.H. Draper of Powell River, and Mrs. F.L. Cassils-Kennedy of Vancouver.

There was, however, one more momentous occasion in his life before he died. On April 29, 1935, he and Beatrice celebrated their golden wedding anniversary, marking 50 years of devotion to their family and their community.

Underhill's death ended a colourful career of great accomplishment. His contribution to Vancouver in its pioneer days is a record that is hard to match. It is unfortunate that Vancouver has never recognized him or his achievements in a tangible way. He is remembered, however, in neighbouring Burnaby, where in 1938 a member of the engineering staff made a recommendation concerning the doctor. Maybe he had survived the flu, or a family member had, or perhaps he recalled that all of the Lower Mainland had benefited from one man's untiring drive, but today there is an Underhill Avenue in Burnaby.

To the end, Dr. Underhill was very much a Victorian-Edwardian, loved by his grandchildren who cheerfully obeyed his

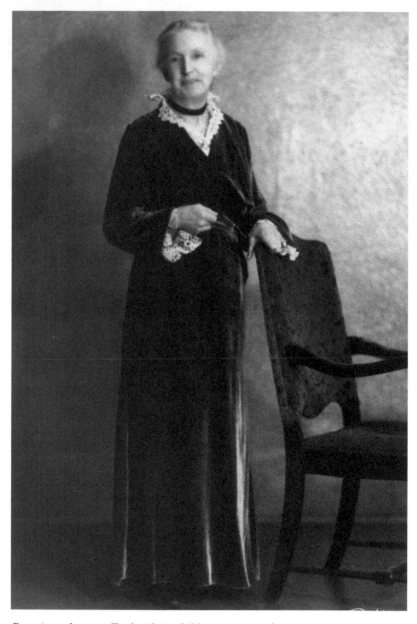

Beatrice, who gave Frederick 13 children, was an adventurous woman with a zest for life and a fondness for gambling. This picture was taken at the time of the couple's 50th wedding anniversary.

code of conduct for the young. One of them, Joan Bryant, recalled years later:

> I remember going into his office, which was in their home. Each one of the grandchildren went in separately—we took turns, usually on the day of the Easter egg hunt or something like that. He looked like King Edward VII, a very proper regal person. You sat on his knee and he said a few words to you, and you said a few words to him, presumably, and then you were dismissed and then the next one came in.
>
> … I remember when I had my tonsils out. I think Ted and I both had them out at the same time. Granddad came in with an entourage of doctors and nurses and gave me a dime and I dropped it behind the crib.

Another granddaughter, Shirley Biehl, remembered going to visit her grandmother, who would let her eat all the ice cream wafers in the apartment. She said Granddad Underhill was always dressed to the nines. "He was always a very portly gentleman," she recalled, "always had a waistcoat on, always a gold watch fob. I can remember he always had a dime for me too."

The woman who was at his side all those years, bearing 13 children in 21 years, sharing the sorrow of the loss of two sons in the First World War, and pulling teeth in the Fraser Valley when her husband was away, survived her husband for 13 years. Beatrice Underhill was 87 when she died on November 14, 1949. She was buried beside her husband in the family plot at Mountain View Cemetery. *The Sun* called her a Vancouver pioneer and mother who proudly watched her children play an active role in the business, sport, and family life of the city. One son, Jack Underhill, was a Canadian badminton champion.

When Beatrice died, she had 29 grandchildren and 16 great-grandchildren. A grandson, Ronald, son of Clare Underhill, served in the RCAF and was killed in action during the Second World War. Ronald's twin sister, Anne Barbara Underhill, died July 3, 2003. She had studied chemistry, physics, and mathematics at UBC and earned a Ph.D. in astrophysics from the University of Chicago; she worked as a professor in Utrecht, The Netherlands, and a scientist with the Goddard Flight Centre in the United States and France. She later returned to Vancouver to serve as honorary professor at UBC.

The Underhill family continues to have a large presence in B.C. Hundreds of them gathered for a family reunion in 1992; among their numbers were the Underhills of Underhill and Underhill Surveyors, a member of the RCMP from Vernon, a chartered accountant from Toronto, as well as educators, lawyers, and army veterans. The last of Fred and Beatrice's children, Enid Anna Kathleen, died in Vancouver in March 1995 at age 96.

☆ ☆ ☆

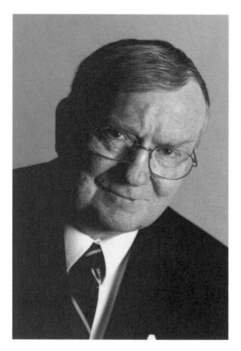

Today, Dr. John Blatherwick, chief medical health officer of the Vancouver Coastal Health Authority, fills the shoes that Underhill did many years ago.

As Dr. Underhill's latest successor, Dr. John Blatherwick hopes he can serve Vancouver nearly as long as the city's first medical health officer did. Underhill was the MHO for 26 years, and after that Dr. Stewart Murray held the post for 22 years: "I am at 19½ years. I won't challenge Dr. Underhill's record, although I will probably pass Stewart Murray. Something about this job says 'stay.' Gerry Bonham, 13 years Vancouver MHO, told me when I took the job, 'Keep it. It is the best job you'll ever have.' I listened."

Dr. Blatherwick's desire for long service will serve his city well. His emphasis on vaccination, particularly for the young and the old, will extend the lives of many, and whether the flu's mysteries are unravelled or remain unknown, the city will get the best advice possible. Following in the steps of the man he very much admires, he echoes his predecessor's oft-repeated advice whenever he gets the chance: "Remember to wash your hands well and frequently."

A verse that ran in the *Illinois Health News* in November 1918 sums up the flu story in a light-hearted way while acknowledging the unanswerable questions:

?Flu?

If we but knew
The cause of flu
And whence it comes and what to do,
I think that you and we folks, too,
Would hardly get in such a stew.
Do you?

REFERENCES

This book is based on original research and interviews. Many newspapers and books were used as information sources; the following were particularly helpful.

Newspapers

The Chilliwack Progress
Comox Argus
The Cranbrook Herald
Cumberland Islander
The Daily Province (Vancouver)
The Daily Colonist (Victoria)
The Edmonton Journal
The Gazette (Montreal)
The Globe and Mail (Toronto)
Kelowna Daily Courier
The Leader-Post (Regina)
Nanaimo Free Press
Nelson Daily News
New Westminster Columbian
The Penticton Herald
Prince George Citizen
Prince Rupert News
The Vancouver Daily Sun
Victoria Daily Times
Winnipeg Free Press

Books

Felicitas, Sister Mary. *The Leaf and the Lamp*. Ottawa: Canadian Nurses' Association, 1968.

Collier, Richard. *The Plague of the Spanish Lady: The Influenza Pandemic of 1918–1919*. London: Macmillan London Ltd., 1974; New York: Atheneum, 1974; London: Allison & Busby, 1996.

Crosby, Alfred W. *Epidemic and Peace, 1918*. Westport, CT: Greenwood Press, 1976. Reprinted as *America's Forgotten Pandemic: The Influenza of 1918*. Cambridge: Cambridge University Press, 1989.

Davies, Pete. *The Devil's Flu: The World's Deadliest Influenza Epidemic and the Scientific Hunt for the Virus That Caused It*. New York: Henry Holt & Company, 2000.

Kolata, Gina. *Flu: The Story of the Great Influenza Pandemic of 1918 and The Search for the Virus that Caused It*. New York: Farrar, Straus, and Giroux, 1999.

Levy, Elinor, and Mark Fischetti. *The New Killer Diseases: How the Alarming Evolution of Germs Threatens Us All*. New York: Crown Publishers, 2003; Random House, 2004.

Pettigrew, Eileen. *The Silent Enemy: Canada and the Deadly Flu of 1918*. Saskatoon: Western Producer Prairie Books, 1983.

PHOTO CREDITS

Front cover photos (clockwise from top left): Dr. Frederick Underhill, courtesy of the Underhill family; nuns who cared for flu victims in Quebec, Archives Soeurs du Bon Pasteur; telephone operators in High River, Alberta, Glenbow Archives (NA-3452-2); influenza poster, Glenbow Archives (NA-4548-5); staff from Ogden Military Hospital in Calgary, Alberta, Glenbow Archives (NA-1721-1). Back cover: Victory Parade on November 11, 1918, in Calgary, Alberta, Glenbow Archives (NC-20-2).

Archives Soeurs du Bon Pasteur: p. 60
Betty O'Keefe and Ian Macdonald: pp. 116, 123, 147
British Columbia Archives: p. 38 (A-02547)
City of Vancouver Archives: pp. 111 (789-56), 129 (Bu PU 550)
Glenbow Archives: pp. 30 (NA-2362-64), 34 (NA-1721-1, Ogden Military Hospital, Calgary, Alberta), 69 (NA-1422-7), 70 (NA-1367-37, top, and NA-2262-10, bottom, R.K. Stickney house in Morrin, Alberta), 72 (NA-964-22, top, and NA-3452-2, bottom), 122 (NA-4548-5), 137 (NA-4230-2, top, Victory parades in Calgary, Alberta, and NA-3965-7, bottom), 139 (NA-3903-95, Victory celebration in the Czechoslovakian community of Frank, Alberta), 155 (NA-1616-1), 179 (NA-521-1, top, and NA-521-8, bottom)
National Archives of Canada: pp. 59 (PA-214115), 120 (PA-025025, Three Men in Rural Alberta), 166 (PA-100229, Windiandy Flats of the Muskeg River, Alberta)

National Museum of Health and Medicine, Armed Forces
    Institute of Pathology (AFIP): pp. 25 (Reeve 15183), 58 (NCP
    1603)
Postcard collection of Fred Thirkell and Bob Scullion: p. 127
St. Paul's Hospital Archives: pp. 78, 97
Underhill family: pp. 41, 42, 44, 46, 48, 53, 75, 205, 206
Vancouver Coastal Health Authority: p. 208
Vancouver Maritime Museum: p. 107
Vancouver Public Library: p. 94 (#3491)
Vancouver School of Theology: p. 101

INDEX

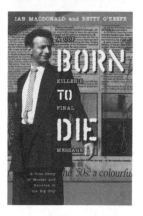
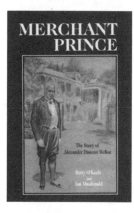
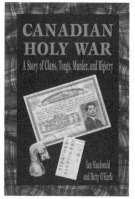

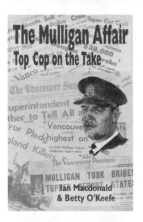
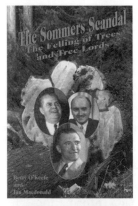
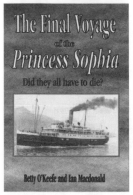

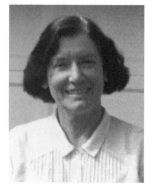
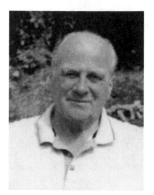

Betty O'Keefe was a Vancouver *Province* reporter for seven years in the 1950s. She worked in corporate communications for 15 years and was commissioned to write two corporate biographies.

After stints at the *The Daily Colonist* (Victoria) and the Vancouver *Province,* Ian Macdonald joined *The Vancouver Sun* and was legislative reporter in Victoria for five years and then bureau chief in Ottawa from 1965 to 1970. He worked in media relations for the prime minister's office and was head of Transport Canada Information. He has written for magazines, radio, television, and film.

Since 1994 Macdonald and O'Keefe have collaborated on writing projects related to West Coast history. Published books include *The Klondike's "Dear Little Nugget"* for Horsdal & Schubart through to 1999's best-seller *The Sommers Scandal. The Mulligan Affair: Top Cop on the Take,* their first book published by Heritage House in 1997, was nominated for the City of Vancouver Book Award. *The Final Voyage of the* Princess Sophia followed in 1998 and *Canadian Holy War* in 2000.